Geriatrics

Editors

DEMETRA ANTIMISIARIS
LAURA MORTON

PRIMARY CARE: CLINICS IN OFFICE PRACTICE

www.primarycare.theclinics.com

Consulting Editor
JOEL J. HEIDELBAUGH

September 2017 • Volume 44 • Number 3

ELSEVIER

1600 John F. Kennedy Boulevard • Suite 1800 • Philadelphia, Pennsylvania, 19103-2899

http://www.theclinics.com

PRIMARY CARE: CLINICS IN OFFICE PRACTICE Volume 44, Number 3
September 2017 ISSN 0095-4543, ISBN-13: 978-0-323-54566-2

Editor: Jessica McCool
Developmental Editor: Colleen Dietzler

Primary Care: Clinics in Office Practice (ISSN: 0095–4543) is published quarterly by Elsevier Inc., 360 Park Avenue South, New York, NY 10010-1710. Months of issue are March, June, September, and December. Periodicals postage paid at New York, NY and additional mailing offices. Subscription prices are $232.00 per year (US individuals), $451.00 (US institutions), $100.00 (US students), $283.00 (Canadian individuals), $511.00 (Canadian institutions), $175.00 (Canadian students), $355.00 (international individuals), $511.00 (international institutions), and $175.00 (international students). Foreign air speed delivery is included in all *Clinics* subscription prices. All prices are subject to change without notice. POSTMASTER: Send address changes to *Primary Care: Clinics in Office Practice*, Elsevier Periodicals Customer Service, 11830 Westline Industrial Drive, St. Louis, MO 63146. Customer Service Health Sciences Division, Subscription Customer Service, 3251 Riverport Lane, Maryland Heights, MO 63043. **Customer Service: 1-800-654-2452 (U.S. and Canada); 314-447-8871 (outside U.S. and Canada). Fax: 314-447-8029. E-mail: journalscustomerservice-usa@elsevier.com (for print support); journalsonlinesupport-usa@elsevier.com (for online support).**

Reprints. For copies of 100 or more, of articles in this publication, please contact the Commercial Reprints Department, Elsevier Inc., 360 Park Avenue South, New York, NY 10010-1710. Tel. 212-633-3874; Fax: 212-633-3820; E-mail: reprints@elsevier.com.

Primary Care: Clinics in Office Practice is covered in *MEDLINE/PubMed (Index Medicus)* and *EMBASE/ Excerpta Medica, Current Contents/Clinical Medicine, and ISI/BIOMED*.

Contributors

CONSULTING EDITOR

JOEL J. HEIDELBAUGH, MD, FAAFP, FACG
Clinical Professor, Departments of Family Medicine and Urology, Director of Medical Student Education and Clerkship Director, Department of Family Medicine, University of Michigan Medical School, Ann Arbor, Michigan; Ypsilanti Health Center, Ypsilanti, Michigan

EDITORS

DEMETRA ANTIMISIARIS, PharmD, BCGP, FASCP
Director, Polypharmacy and Medication Management Program, Associate Professor, Departments of Pharmacology and Toxicology, Neurology, and Family and Geriatric Medicine, University of Louisville, School of Medicine, Louisville, Kentucky

LAURA MORTON, MD, CMD
Assistant Professor, Department of Family and Geriatric Medicine, University of Louisville School of Medicine, Louisville, Kentucky

AUTHORS

DEMETRA ANTIMISIARIS, PharmD, BCGP, FASCP
Director, Polypharmacy and Medication Management Program, Associate Professor, Departments of Pharmacology and Toxicology, Neurology, and Family and Geriatric Medicine, University of Louisville School of Medicine, Louisville, Kentucky

ELIZABETH AUBREY BROWN, MD
The Donald W. Reynolds Department of Geriatric Medicine, University of Oklahoma Health Sciences Center, College of Medicine, Hospice and Palliative Care Fellow, Oklahoma City VA Medical Center, Oklahoma City, Oklahoma

DAVID A. CASEY, MD
Professor and Chair, Chief of the Geriatric Psychiatry Program, Department of Psychiatry and Behavioral Sciences, University of Louisville School of Medicine, Louisville, Kentucky

JANET SOOJEUNG CHO, PharmD, CDE, BCGP
USC Specialty Pharmacy, University of Southern California, School of Pharmacy, Alhambra, California

TIMOTHY CUTLER, PharmD, BCGP
Professor, Department of Clinical Pharmacy, University of California, San Francisco School of Pharmacy, San Francisco, California

LUCIA LOREDANA DATTOMA, MD
Associate Clinical Professor, Division of Geriatrics, Department of Medicine, David Geffen School of Medicine at UCLA, Simi Valley, California

ANDREW DENTINO, MD, FACP, AGSF, FAPA, FAAHPM
Professor and Chairman, The Donald W. Reynolds Department of Geriatric Medicine, The University of Oklahoma Health Sciences Center, College of Medicine, Oklahoma City, Oklahoma

RANGARAJ GOPALRAJ, MD, PhD
Assistant Professor, Department of Family and Geriatric Medicine, University of Louisville, School of Medicine, Louisville, Kentucky

HOLLY M. HOLMES, MD, MS, AGSF
Division Director, Geriatric and Palliative Medicine, Associate Professor, Department of Internal Medicine, University of Texas Houston McGovern Medical School, Houston, Texas

GREGORY JICHA, MD, PhD
Professor, Department of Neurology, University of Kentucky, Lexington, Kentucky

SUSAN D. LEONARD, MD
Assistant Clinical Professor, Division of Geriatrics, University of California, Los Angeles, Los Angeles, California

STEFANI MADISON, MD
Assistant Professor, Hospice and Palliative Medicine, Physician, Denver Health, Denver, Colorado

ROBERTO MEDINA, MD
Donald W. Reynolds Department of Geriatric Medicine, The University of Oklahoma Health Sciences Center, College of Medicine, Oklahoma City, Oklahoma

DANIELA CLAUDIA MOGA, MD, PhD
Assistant Professor, Department of Pharmacy Practice and Science, College of Pharmacy, Department of Epidemiology, College of Public Health, University of Kentucky, Lexington, Kentucky

LAURA MORTON, MD, CMD
Assistant Professor, Department of Family and Geriatric Medicine, University of Louisville School of Medicine, Louisville, Kentucky

MONICA ROBERTS, PharmD
College of Pharmacy, University of Kentucky, Lexington, Kentucky

BELINDA SETTERS, MD, MS, AGSF, FACP
Director, Inpatient Geriatrics, Robley Rex VA Medical Center, Associate Professor, Departments of Internal Medicine and Family and Geriatric Medicine, University of Louisville School of Medicine, Louisville, Kentucky

LAURENCE M. SOLBERG, MD, AGSF
Ruth S. Jewett Professor of Geriatric Medicine, Chief, Division of Geriatric Medicine, Department of Aging and Geriatric Research, University of Florida College of Medicine, Geriatrician, GRECC, Malcom Randall VA Medical Center, Gainesville, Florida

EUGENE STEINBERG, MD
The Donald W. Reynolds Department of Geriatric Medicine, The University of Oklahoma Health Sciences Center College of Medicine, Oklahoma City, Oklahoma

BRYAN DAVID STRUCK, MD
Medical Director, Hospice and Palliative Care Medicine, Oklahoma City VA Medical Center, Associate Professor, The Donald W. Reynolds Department of Geriatric Medicine, University of Oklahoma Health Sciences Center College of Medicine, Oklahoma City, Oklahoma

HONG-PHUC T. TRAN, MD
Assistant Clinical Professor, Division of Geriatrics, University of California, Los Angeles, Los Angeles, California

BRADLEY R. WILLIAMS, PharmD, BCGP
Titus Family Department of Clinical Pharmacy, University of Southern California, School of Pharmacy, Los Angeles, California

Contents

> Because of a growing, aging population and a shortage of geriatricians in the United States, the care of geriatric patients will mostly devolve to primary care providers. This article reviews the different aspects of a multidimensional, multidisciplinary geriatric assessment. Assessment tools and training of office staff to take on larger roles can help primary care providers reduce the burden of work associated with performing a comprehensive geriatric assessment.

> Polypharmacy is an underappreciated factor in undesirable patient outcomes. In older adults, polypharmacy is considered a syndrome of harm and presents a challenge to primary care providers. The United States has one of the highest medication use rates per capita in the world. With the aging population, and polypharmacy a significant part of the lives of older adults, management of polypharmacy poses both a growing challenge and an opportunity for all health care providers. This article provides an overview of skills to improve medication use management in older adults living with polypharmacy.

> Sexuality is an important part of a person's life continuing into older age. Physiologic changes that occur with aging can affect sexual function and may be exacerbated by comorbid disease. To diagnose sexual dysfunction, providers must obtain a thorough history and physical examination, including psychosocial factors. The causes of sexual dysfunction along with patient preferences within the patient's social system serve as the foundation for developing person-centered strategies to address these concerns. To improve care of older adults with sexual concerns, providers should initiate discussions with, listen to, and work with patients to create a comprehensive management plan.

Dementia represents one of the most important and growing public health issues facing society today. Primary care clinics serve a crucial role as the first line of defense in the recognition and treatment of dementia. Increased awareness and treatment of risk factors for dementia are important for lessening disease burden in the population. Diagnostic workup should include screening for medical and nondegenerative causes of cognitive impairment that may be remedial. Treatment approaches should include multimodal approaches to address cognitive decline and behavioral/psychiatric symptoms of dementia in an effort to maximize quality of life for both patients and caregivers.

Older adults in the United States are healthier and more active than ever before. The number of adult drivers 65 years and older is increasing rapidly. However, older drivers are involved in more fatal car incidents per miles driven than any other age group except teenagers. Driving has become very important for older adults because it is critical to their independence and self-esteem. Therefore, the role of health care providers and the interprofessional team is essential to maximizing the life expectancy of driving to match the life span and activity levels of the older adult population.

Busy primary care providers are in the frontline and see the bulk of older adults with diabetes. This vulnerable population is more prone to diabetic complications and hypoglycemia. In contrast to the younger patients with diabetes, lifestyle interventions are even more effective in older adults while the target A1c levels may need to be more relaxed for frail individuals. Geriatric syndromes can adversely affect diabetes care. A team with experts in different fields who understand the needs of older adults is essential for the adequate quality care of the whole individual with diabetes.

Natural aging brings reduced production of growth and sex hormones, beginning in middle age, with noticeable physiologic changes by the sixth or seventh decade of life: reduced muscle mass, energy, and exercise capacity and alterations in sexual function. Hormones and hormone precursors have been investigated to delay changes in body composition, strength, and physical and cognitive function. Menopausal hormone therapy is effective for vasomotor and genitourinary symptoms. Testosterone is effective in men with hypogonadism and declines in physiologic function. The lack of clinical studies evaluating the long-term effects and risks of hormone replacement limits its use.

considered a diagnosis reserved for the hospital setting. However, delirium is known to occur as both an acute and subacute condition that carries significant morbidity and mortality. The association of delirium with dementia and aging makes delirium an important topic for primary care providers to become more familiar with as they are tasked with caring for an aging population.

PRIMARY CARE:
CLINICS IN OFFICE PRACTICE

ISSUE OF RELATED INTEREST

Clinics in Geriatric Medicine, November 2016 (Vol. 32, Issue 4)
Geriatric Pain Management
M. Carrington Reid, *Editor*
http://www.geriatric.theclinics.com/

THE CLINICS ARE AVAILABLE ONLINE!
Access your subscription at:
www.theclinics.com

PRIMARY CARE:
CLINICS IN OFFICE PRACTICE

FORTHCOMING ISSUES

December 2017
Gastroenterology
Rick Kellerman and Laura Mayans,
Editors

March 2018
Cardiovascular Disease
Mark Stephens, Editor

June 2018
Rheumatology
Seetha Monrad and Daniel F. Battafarano,
Editors

RECENT ISSUES

June 2017
Integrative Medicine
Deborah S. Clements and Melinda Ring,
Editors

March 2017
Primary Care of the Medically Underserved
Vincent Morelli, Roger Zoorob, and
Joel J. Heidelbaugh, Editors

December 2016
Hematologic Diseases
Maureen Okam Achebe and Aric Parnes,
Editors

ISSUE OF RELATED INTEREST

Clinics in Geriatric Medicine November 2016 (Vol. 32, Issue 4)
Geriatric Pain Management
M. Carrington Reid, Editor
(http://www.geriatric.theclinics.com/)

THE CLINICS ARE AVAILABLE ONLINE!
Access your subscription at:
www.theclinics.com

Foreword
The Art of Managing Complexity, The Joy of Aging Gracefully

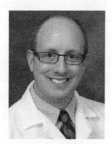

Joel J. Heidelbaugh, MD, FAAFP, FACG
Consulting Editor

As a medical educator in family medicine, I am often asked by my students and residents, *"Why do they make you see so many patients per day"*? While I strive not to base my days upon productivity requirements and statistics (wishful thinking…), perhaps the more appropriate questions should be, *"How many issues do you address per visit with your older patients?"*, or *"How long does it take to perform medication reconciliation on a geriatric patient?"* There is currently a national shortage of primary care providers trained in care of the geriatric patient, and as the population ages, that shortage will certainly grow. These shortages are more pronounced in suburban and rural areas. The next generation of health care providers continues to gravitate toward subspecialty and procedure-based care, likely due to higher reimbursement, and somewhat different challenges of patient complexity. This trend in the workforce will need to change quickly, or the geriatric patients risk becoming an underserved population in primary care.

Many patients are in search of the fountain of youth, and some want to capitalize on the latest supplements and technologies to delay aging. In a recent visit with a 77-year-old woman and her two middle-aged sons, her chief concerns included how to get a prescription for antiaging hormones, how to improve her libido, and how to appear younger. Much to the surprise of her sons, she had engaged in plentiful Internet "research" on various therapies for these concerns. In particular, she was interested in lengthening her telomeres, getting stem cell therapy for her arthritis, and getting a prescription for human chorionic gonadotropin to "rewind the clock."

While geriatric patients are often complex from medical and psychosocial standpoints, I find the care of this patient population to be very rewarding and endearing. Geriatric patients have amazing perspectives on life, death, family, and even the evolution of health care. Providing advice on day-to-day living for geriatric patients with consultation of patients' families can be a unique challenge. This can include giving

Prim Care Clin Office Pract 44 (2017) xiii–xiv
http://dx.doi.org/10.1016/j.pop.2017.06.002
0095-4543/17/© 2017 Published by Elsevier Inc.

recommendations on ambulation, driving, administration of medications, and managing finances. Often, these are challenging discussions that we must mediate with patients and families, for the benefit of the safety of the patient. Depression, dementia, delirium, mental illness, and pain often go underevaluated and undiagnosed. Discussions centered on advanced care planning also present challenges that affect patient autonomy and finances.

I sincerely thank Drs Antimisiaris and Morton for their brilliant efforts in compiling this timely issue on the care of the geriatric patient. Moreover, I thank their dedicated authors for their substantial efforts in compiling a very practical issue of the *Primary Care: Clinics in Office Practice* centered on the care of the geriatric patient. The articles within this issue address the aforementioned topics and provide current strategies for improving morbidity, mortality, and wellness of our elder patients. I hope that our readers will benefit from this knowledge, master the art of managing complex elder patients, and guide them toward aging gracefully.

Joel J. Heidelbaugh, MD, FAAFP, FACG
Departments of Family Medicine and Urology
University of Michigan Medical School
Ann Arbor, MI 48103, USA

Ypsilanti Health Center
200 Arnet, Suite 200
Ypsilanti, MI 48198, USA

E-mail address:
jheidel@umich.edu

Preface
The Urgent Need for Robust Geriatric Patient Care Skills in Primary Care

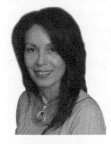 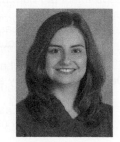

Demetra Antimisiaris,   Laura Morton, MD, CMD
PharmD, BCGP, FASCP
                    Editors

The world's population, including in the United States, is aging at an exponential rate. Currently, there are only 7,293 allopathic and osteopathic certified geriatricians in the United States (6,928 in allopathic medicine and 365 osteopathic medicine). This translates to 1 geriatrician for every 2,725 Americans over 75 years old. With the projected increase in the number of older Americans, the aging workforce and retirement of many geriatricians, and plateau in the number of geriatricians over the last 10 years, this ratio is expected to change to 1 geriatrician for every 4,567 older Americans in 2030. In terms of geropsychiatrists, there are currently 1,544 (1,531 allopathic and 13 osteopathic), or 1 for every 12,869 older Americans, and is projected to decrease to 1 geropsychiatrist for every 21,573 Americans over the age of 75 by 2030.[1–3]

Presently, there are not enough graduating geriatricians to replace the geriatricians going into retirement, let alone provide care for the country's growing elderly population. Based on the continued shortages of geriatricians, *it appears that primary care physicians* will bear the responsibility for caring for most of the elderly.[3] However, geriatric content has not been a focal point in undergraduate medical education, and minimum requirements for geriatric competency tend to be lacking.[4,5]

This issue of *Primary Care: Clinics in Office Practice* provides primary care providers with resources and a review of topics that the authors and editors believe can be useful in day-to-day care of older adult patients. Many of the problems encountered in providing care for the older adult require interpretation of guidelines for the individual patient living with complex medical, functional, and psychosocial challenges. The care of older adults requires comprehensive assessment and solutions for medical, functional, social, environmental, and legal challenges. Although older adult patients are

Prim Care Clin Office Pract 44 (2017) xv–xvi
http://dx.doi.org/10.1016/j.pop.2017.06.001
0095-4543/17/© 2017 Published by Elsevier Inc.

complex to manage, the return on investment for robust comprehensive geriatric patient management skills is significant, ranging from avoided hospitalizations and improved quality measures to the satisfaction that we are providing high-quality care for an aging society.[6] We hope you will find this compilation of topics written by Geriatrics experts useful and valuable for your practice.

Demetra Antimisiaris, PharmD, BCGP, FASCP
University of Louisville Polypharmacy
and Medication Management Program
Department of Pharmacology and Toxicology
Department of Family Medicine and Geriatrics
501 East Broadway, Suite 240
Louisville, KY 40202, USA

Laura Morton, MD, CMD
Department of Family and Geriatric Medicine
University of Louisville
501 East Broadway, Suite 240
Louisville, KY 40202, USA

E-mail addresses:
demetra.antimisiaris@louisville.edu (D. Antimisiaris)
Laura.Morton@louisville.edu (L. Morton)

REFERENCES

1. 2015-2016 ABMS Board Certification Report. Geographic Distribution of ABMS Member Board Diplomates by Subspecialty Certification. 2016. Available at: http://www.abms.org/media/131568/2015-16-abmscertreport.pdf. Accessed April 1, 2017.
2. Scheinthal S, Kramer J, Marales-Egizi L. Appendix 2: American Osteopathic Association Specialty Board Certification. J Am Osteopath Assoc 2016;116(4):263–6.
3. AGS Web site. Advocacy Public Policy section. Available at: http://www.americangeriatrics.org/advocacy_public_policy/gwps/gwps_faqs/. Accessed April 1, 2017.
4. Gawande A. Annals of Medicine: The Way We Age Now. The New Yorker 2007. Available at: http://www.newyorker.com/magazine/2007/04/30/the-way-we-age-now. Accessed April 1, 2017.
5. Eleazer GP, Brummel-Smith K. Commentary: Aging America: meeting the needs of older Americans and the crisis in geriatrics. Acad Med 2009;84(5):542–4. Available at: http://journals.lww.com/academicmedicine/Fulltext/2009/05000/Commentary__Aging_America__Meeting_the_Needs_of.4.aspx. Accessed April 1, 2017.
6. Available at: http://www.thescanfoundation.org/sites/thescanfoundation.org/files/achieving_positive_roi_fact_sheet_3_0.pdf. Accessed April 1, 2017.

Geriatric Assessment for Primary Care Providers

Hong-Phuc T. Tran, MD[a],*, Susan D. Leonard, MD[b]

KEYWORDS

- Geriatric • Assessment • Function • Elder • Geriatric syndrome • Older adult

KEY POINTS

- Cognitive deficits, delirium, functional decline, falls, incontinence, pressure ulcers, and frailty are examples of geriatric syndromes.
- A comprehensive geriatric assessment evaluates multiple domains, including social, functional, economic, psychosocial, cognitive, and environmental, and uses interdisciplinary teams to develop a coordinated plan of care for the older adult.
- In the geriatric population, the initial sign of a medical problem may be a change or decline in function and mental status, rather than a clinical or laboratory abnormality.
- Assessment tools can help reduce the burden of work in performing comprehensive geriatric assessments; additionally, office staff can be trained to take larger roles in assessing and monitoring older adults.

INTRODUCTION

Because of a growing, aging population and worsening shortage of geriatricians in the United States, the care of geriatric patients will mostly devolve to primary care providers. In 2004, there was an estimated 1 fellowship-trained geriatrician for every 10,350 Americans aged 75 years and older.[1] Hence, it is imperative that primary care providers be trained and comfortable with managing geriatric syndromes and multiple chronic medical conditions, as well as delivering high-quality, cost-effective care to the elderly. In 2011, the first cohort of the American baby boomers (those born between 1945 and 1966) reached age 65 years and, by 2030, 1 in every 5 Americans will be 65 years of age and older.[1] Medicare beneficiaries with 4 or more chronic conditions generate 80% of all Medicare spending.[1] Preparing primary care physicians to provide expert geriatric chronic care and increasing the workforce of primary care physicians can help older adults receive better access to skilled providers and

Conflicts of interest: The authors have no conflicts of interest to report.
[a] Division of Geriatrics, UCLA, 1223 16th Street, Suite 3100, Los Angeles, CA, USA; [b] Division of Geriatrics, UCLA, 200 Medical Plaza, Suite 365-A, Los Angeles, CA 90095, USA
* Corresponding author.
E-mail address: hongphuctran@mednet.ucla.edu

Prim Care Clin Office Pract 44 (2017) 399–411
http://dx.doi.org/10.1016/j.pop.2017.05.001
0095-4543/17/© 2017 Elsevier Inc. All rights reserved.

help improve the Medicare budgetary crisis. This article focuses on geriatric assessment for primary care providers.

MULTIFACTORIAL AND MULTIDISCIPLINARY APPROACH

The geriatric medical assessment is an important diagnostic tool to use while assessing the elderly. Older individuals may have more comorbidities and impairments that contribute to functional decline, and recognizing how various disciplines work together to affect outcome can guide decision making and medical management. The assessment goes beyond just medical conditions to include a spectrum of systems including social, functional, economic, psychosocial, cognitive, and environmental conditions.[2] Ranging from brief screens to more extensive evaluations, the geriatric assessment addresses how the domains interplay to affect functional status.

The functional evaluation is a fundamental concept in the framework of the geriatric assessment. Functional status can be seen as a measure of overall health impact in the context of an individual's environment and social support network. As individuals live longer, they survive longer with functional impairments. In the geriatric population, the initial sign of a medical problem may be a decline or change in function rather than a clinical abnormality. Effective medical management accounts for overall function instead of management of acute symptoms.

PHYSICAL HEALTH AND INTRODUCTION TO GERIATRIC SYNDROMES

When assessing the physical health of geriatric patients, different components need to be taken into account, such as acute and chronic medical issues, vision and hearing, continence, nutrition, gait, and sleep disorders.

Geriatric syndrome is a term used to describe unique health conditions in elderly patients that are multifactorial in cause and do not fit into discrete organ-based categories. Examples of geriatric syndromes include functional decline, falls, frailty, incontinence, and pressure ulcers.[3] Cognitive deficits and delirium are geriatric syndromes that are discussed elsewhere in this issue. Frailty is an impairment in mobility, balance, endurance, physical activity, muscle strength, nutrition, and cognition; it is the overarching geriatric syndrome.[3] The constellation of other geriatric syndromes (such as falls, delirium, functional decline, and/or pressure ulcers) can lead to frailty, and frailty itself can feed back to result in the development of more risk factors and, in turn, even more geriatric syndromes, with the final outcomes being disability, dependence, and death.[3]

MEDICAL

Primary care providers need to be adept at diagnosing and managing the geriatric syndromes (mentioned earlier) and common medical conditions in older adults. The geriatric assessment should be comprehensive and holistic; however, time constraints may limit the realistic ability to perform thorough evaluations. The medical assessment of older adults can be done by physicians, nurse practitioners, or physician assistants; efficiency in the office visit can be achieved by using medical assistants and/or nurses to help with data gathering and performing standardized assessments.

Older adults often present with vague complaints, such as dizziness, and may have cognitive deficits that affect their ability to provide a concise, accurate history. They may under-report or over-report symptoms. In a brief office encounter, it may be difficult to obtain all the relevant details in a timely manner. Hence, eliciting collateral information from the patient's family or caregivers can greatly help the primary care provider in making a diagnostic evaluation. For older adults with cognitive deficits who come to their appointments alone, the primary care provider can consider calling the family or caregiver to "attend" the interview portion of the visit via telephone conference. If a geriatric patient lives in an assisted-living or board-and-care facility, contacting the facility for an updated medication list and collateral information is helpful. Previsit and self-report questionnaires can also help with information gathering and can be done by trained office staff. Medication reconciliation can also be performed by office staff.

VISION AND HEARING

Sensory deficits can greatly affect the quality of life of older adults. About 16% of adults 75 to 84 years old and 27% of those 85 years of age and older are unable to read newsprint (even with correction lenses). Cataracts, age-related macular degeneration, and glaucoma are common causes of vision problems in older adults. Vision loss is a risk factor for hip fractures and motor-vehicle accidents and is associated with faster physical decline and greater mortality. Screening for (and correcting) vision loss may prevent these effects.[4] The Snellen eye chart is a quick way to assess vision.

Age-related sensorineural hearing loss is a common problem in geriatric patients, and can lead to social isolation, depression, and reduced quality of life. Presbycusis is the most common cause of hearing loss, and is the progressive decline in ability to perceive high-frequency tones, caused by degeneration of hair cells in the ear. Hearing loss is associated with falls, cognitive and physical decline, and increased mortality. The Whisper test, finger rub, or handheld audiometer can be used to assess hearing and can be done by office staff. For patients with moderate to severe hearing deficits, a pocket-talker (see https://www.hearingspeech.org/services/hearing-aids/assistive-listening-devices/) can be used to amplify sound and help patients hear, potentially making the office visit more efficient. Referrals to audiologists for further hearing evaluation and assessment for hearing aids can be made if indicated.[5]

URINARY INCONTINENCE

Urine incontinence is a common source of emotional distress and embarrassment for older adults and can lead to social isolation. Despite being common, many community-dwelling older adults with urinary incontinence, especially women, do not seek help from their medical providers.[6] The presence of urine incontinence can be assessed with brief screening questionnaires, postvoid residual (if bladder scanner is available), and urine dipstick. A postvoid residual can assist with determining whether urine retention is contributing to overflow urinary incontinence. A urine dipstick can help rule out a urinary tract infection. In older adults using multiple medications, assessment of medications and their potential contributions to urinary incontinence should be performed (for a review and resources regarding the assessment of urinary incontinence see http://www.aafp.org/afp/2013/0415/p543.html#afp20130415p543-f1). Patient resources can be found at the National Association for Continence (see https://www.nafc.org/urinary-incontinence/).

NUTRITION

Nutritional status in older adults is determined by multiple factors, such as comorbid medical conditions, activity level, energy expenditure, and caloric requirements. The ability to access, prepare, ingest, and digest food, and also appetite, are important considerations. Nutrition can be assessed by weight, height, and body mass index.

Because of decreased physiologic reserves associated with increasing age, older adults are at increased risk of malnutrition, especially after an acute illness or hospitalization. There are various criteria for clinically significant weight loss; the Centers for Medicare and Medicaid Services' Resident Assessment Instrument (RAI) Minimum Data Set (MDS) Version 3.0 uses the proposed criteria of weight loss of 5% or greater of baseline body weight in 30 days, or 10% or more of baseline body weight in 6 months for nursing facility patients (see https://www.cms.gov/Medicare/Quality-Initiatives-Patient-Assessment-Instruments/NursingHomeQualityInits/Downloads/MDS-30-RAI-Manual-V113.pdf).

For patients with significant weight loss, it is important to assess psychological, socioeconomic, and cognitive factors that may be contributing to the older patient's nutritional decline. For example, cognitive decline can lead to swallowing difficulties and depression may lead to anorexia. A social worker on the interdisciplinary team can help assess the older patient's living situation and available resources. Similarly, a psychologist on the team can help with psychotherapy and management of depression and other mood disorders. Meal delivery services, such as Meals on Wheels or local delivery programs, can help improve accessibility to food. The Area Agencies on Aging (see https://www.n4a.org/aaastitlevi) can help patients access services geared toward aging in place, and Meals on Wheels is one such service. Nutritional supplements, such as protein shakes, offered 1 to 3 times daily can help older adults gain weight. After a thorough review of the patient's medications and medical, socioeconomic, and psychological history, the medical provider can devise a plan of care that suits the needs and goals of the patient. Appetite stimulants can also be considered if indicated. Keep in mind that megestrol is listed as a Beers Criterion (see http://onlinelibrary.wiley.com/doi/10.1111/jgs.13702/pdf) potentially inappropriate medication in the elderly because it can increase risk of cardiovascular thrombi and is of controversial efficacy. Mirtazapine is also used to stimulate appetite, and that effect is typically observed with low-dose use, at which level the drug has primarily antihistaminic activity (at higher doses it has increased serotonergic activity).[7]

SLEEP

Changes in sleep are a normal part of aging; however, they can be problematic for older adults who consider good sleep important to quality of life. Common sleep complaints include difficulty falling asleep, nighttime awakening, early morning awakening, and daytime sleepiness. Risk factors associated with sleep disorders include underlying mood disorder, dementia, comorbid medical conditions, and use of multiple medications.[8,9]

Assessment of sleep in older adults should include the following elements:

- Typical bedtime and rise time on weekdays and weekends
- Presence of daily sleep routine or ritual (eg, what does the patient do before going to sleep?)
- Difficulty falling or staying asleep or both
- Presence and frequency of daytime naps and their duration
- Quality of sleep (eg, does the patient feel refreshed after waking up after a night's sleep? How many times does the patient wake up during sleep? How long does it take for patient to fall back to sleep?)
- Presence of snoring or apnea
- Presence of restless legs syndrome
- Presence of daytime drowsiness or fatigue
- Presence or absence of shift work

- Activities that are affected by poor sleep
- Use of sleep aids
- Presence of depression

Assessment of sleep disorders should also include a thorough review of the patient's medications to identify any possible causes (eg, if a patient is on diuretics, is the patient taking the diuretic in the afternoon or evening?). A sleep diary detailing these elements is helpful in assessing for the presence of a sleep disorder. The consensus sleep diary, which is a standard sleep diary developed by a panel of insomnia experts, can be given to patients to complete and can be used to assess for sleep disorders; there are 3 different versions of the consensus sleep diary (with different formatting/charts) available for medical providers to use. In a busy clinic practice, time can be saved by giving a sleep diary to patients or their families to complete and having the patient return to discuss the findings in the sleep diary and treatment recommendations.[10]

Encouraging behavioral measures, such as good sleep hygiene, is key to improving sleep. Features of good sleep hygiene include minimizing daytime naps, keeping a regular bedtime and routine of relaxation, avoiding television in bed, and minimizing excessive fluid intake a few hours before bedtime. Hypnotics (benzodiazepines, non-benzodiazepines, anticholinergics like tricyclic antidepressants, and antihistamines like diphenhydramine) should be avoided because they carry increased risk of confusion, delirium, falls, and adverse side effects.[11]

MEDICATIONS AND POLYPHARMACY

A thorough review of medication adverse side effects, drug-drug interactions, and medication adherence is crucial in determining whether medications are contributing to a patient's symptoms or functional impairment. Office staff can be trained to assist with medication reconciliation and medication refills. The topic of polypharmacy is further discussed elsewhere in this issue.

FUNCTIONAL ASSESSMENT

Activities of daily living (ADLs) are used to assess function in elderly. These are divided into 3 levels: basic activities of daily living (BADLs; commonly referred to as simply ADLs), instrumental ADLs (IADLs), and advanced ADLs (AADLs).

BADLs are self-care activities that an individual must accomplish in order to survive self-sufficiently. These activities include bathing, dressing, toileting, transferring, maintaining continence, and feeding. Patients tend to lose these abilities in this order, and regain them in the opposite order during rehabilitation. Inability to perform these tasks indicates the need for additional caregiver assistance or placement into a higher level of care.

IADLs are higher-level activities that an individual must perform or have help with in order to remain independent in their living environments. These activities include using the telephone, shopping, doing housework, doing laundry, preparing meals, driving, taking medications, and managing money. Dependency in IADLs is more common and the progressive loss of more IADL functions translates to more difficulty remaining independent in the household. Some social services are available to provide assistance with these needs, such as meal delivery and transportation services. Assisted living facilities can provide help with IADLs, but usually not for BADLs unless for an additional cost.

The clinical implications are important because ADL impairment can lead to functional decline, decreased quality of life, and loss of independence. Furthermore, it can affect prognosis and hospital outcomes, and predict morbidity and mortality.[12] Early intervention through detection of functional decline leads to reductions in negative outcomes. Changes in functional activity can also be a stronger predictor than admitting diagnoses, and other indices of illness burden. Many older patients lose some aspect of function or independence in their ADLs after being hospitalized.[12] Some risk factors include IADL impairments before admission, advanced age, and preexisting cognitive impairment.[13,14]

AADLs are more advanced tasks require a higher level of understanding and integration into societal and community roles. Examples include occupational, recreational, and travel activities. A decline in the ability to perform such tasks is often the first sign of functional change before disability.

Furthermore, understanding baseline function provides insight into setting appropriate expectations and goals. Older adults who are hospitalized should be asked about their functional status before admission to compare with the level of function at the time of discharge. Individuals in the nursing home generally depend on their IADLs, so assessing ADL capabilities becomes more relevant.

A previsit questionnaire can be helpful in making such assessments, staying mindful that most answers are by self or proxy (informant such as caregiver, family, friend) report and may have intrinsic variability. Having such questionnaires completed in advance saves time and also provides insight into the individual's concerns and cognitive ability. The Lawton IADL and Katz ADL questionnaires (see https://clas.uiowa.edu/socialwork/sites/clas.uiowa.edu.socialwork/files/NursingHomeResource/documents/Katz%20ADL_LawtonIADL.pdf) are standard screening tools for ADL and IADLs.

Many individuals tend to over-report their abilities, whereas family members may under-report abilities. Evaluation from physical and occupational therapists can provide a more objective perspective on a person's capabilities and help guide rehabilitation goals and care needs.

Functional status is essential as a basis for following the progress of patients with chronic disabilities. The functional assessment can provide valuable prognostic information to direct appropriate diagnostic evaluation, treatment plans, and goal discussions. Changes or losses in function should be understood in a context beyond just the medical conditions, and should address the environmental and social supports that interplay to affect older people's needs and goals.

GAIT AND MOBILITY ASSESSMENT

Fall-related injuries are associated with decline in functional status, increased morbidity and mortality, and increased likelihood of nursing home placement.[15] The ability to get up after a fall and the fear of falling are associated with worse outcomes and increased risk of institutionalization.

The timed Get Up and Go test can be used to screen gait, balance, and mobility in older adults. In this test, the patient is asked to rise from a standard arm chair, walk 3 m (10 feet) across the room, turn around, walk back to the chair, and sit down. More than 16 seconds to complete this test suggest an increased risk of falling, functional decline, and poor health.[16] Time-saving measures can be achieved by having office staff perform the Get up and Go test. Gait and mobility assessment can help identify older adults who would benefit from assistive devices, such as cane or walker, and physical therapy. Gait, balance, and strengthening exercises can help minimize risk of falls in older adults. Older adults who need to be lifted or who require more than 1 person's assistance to move can rarely be accommodated in their own homes; they may need hired caregivers to remain living in their own homes or placement in assisted living facilities or nursing homes where additional support staff are available.

SOCIAL/ENVIRONMENTAL ASSESSMENT

The well-being of the elderly is greatly influenced by social conditions, more so than other age groups. Because so much of elderly health is affected by the patients' social environments and support networks, sufficient understanding of the social history is necessary to provide effective patient care. Knowing the main source of support at home may include involvement of family, friends, or outside assistance for caregiving. It is also important to recognize the individual's personal values, preferences, and goals, and (more importantly) whether these goals are realistic in the context of the patient's functional status.

The social history should involve asking about the living environment and home safety, support structure, family relationships, education, habits, caregiving needs, exercise, community involvement, and advanced care planning. Other important questions include addressing financial security, safety, and injury risk.

Understanding an elderly person's living conditions can give insight into that person's overall health status. Many seniors want to remain in their own home environment. However, the living environment may be unsafe or be a leading area of injury from falls. Falls are common in the elderly and contribute to loss of independence and increased morbidity and mortality.

Home safety evaluation can reveal many high-risk conditions and correcting these can improve the home setting. Some hazards can be quickly corrected, whereas others may require more substantial home modification or prompt changing into a different environment or higher level of care. Usually home safety evaluations can be conducted by home health from a physical or occupational therapist.

Understanding the social support and caregiving status is critical in the older population. Adequate care is necessary for safety at home. Caregivers should be screened for caregiver burnout and, if concerned, referred to support groups or work on alternative caregiving arrangements.

It is important to assess for basic habits and behaviors, including tobacco, alcohol, and substance abuse in the elderly, because these may not be obvious. Habits have an effect on health outcomes, especially those that have accumulated over decades. Mortality can be delayed even in smokers who quit after the age of 70 years. Substance abuse cessation is encouraged in the elderly.

Exercise can have numerous beneficial effects and can improve cardiovascular and cerebrovascular health, decrease pain, and improve mortality. It also improves balance, flexibility, fitness, mood, sleep, and cognition. Information on physical activity and status on a patient can help prognosticate functional outcomes.

Sexual activity and health remain relevant in the elderly. Sexually transmitted diseases and human immunodeficiency virus are increasing in the older population and it is important to ask the necessary questions. Similarly, many people are concerned about the opposite problem: sexual dysfunction. Impotence and sexual dysfunction are often not discussed easily, although they are common. It is important to obtain the relevant information in the history to discuss potential treatment options.

Furthermore, elder mistreatment is a topic that should not be overlooked. The National Research Council defines mistreatment of older adults as "intentional actions that cause harm or create a serious risk of harm (whether or not harm is intended) to a vulnerable elder by a caregiver or other person who stands in a trust relationship to the elder. This includes failure by a caregiver to satisfy the elder's basic needs or to protect the elder from harm."[17] Risk factors for mistreatment of older adults include poverty, functional disability and dependency, frailty, and cognitive impairment. Elder mistreatment should also be screened, especially if there are concerns about suspicious skin marks, contusions, trauma, ulcers, malnutrition, or poor care without explanation. In addition to physical consequences, other forms of mistreatment include psychological mistreatment, neglect, and financial exploitation. Clinicians are in a key position to evaluate and report suspected elder abuse and mistreatment. Support for interventions can include assistance from social work staff and state adult protective services (www.napsa-now.org).

RESIDENTIAL LIVING OPTIONS AND LEVELS OF CARE

- A major question that frequently arises is whether the older person is in the right living environment, which must balance respect for a person's autonomy and independence with concerns about safety.
- Older people who do not have adequate support or the ability to live in their own homes may need to consider residential long-term settings, and a range of options are available depending on needs and resources.
- Residential care communities can be divided into several categories. Independent living facilities are senior living homes in a complex that offers recreational activities but still requires the individuals to be independent with ADLs.
- Assisted living facilities (ALFs) are options for individuals who need additional assistance with ADLs but not skilled nursing care. Services provided may include administration or supervision of medications and help with personal care, usually for an additional fee. ALFs are paid for privately, although there may be limited coverage from Medicaid and waiver programs.
- Board-and-care facilities offer a house-style living environment that houses approximately 4 to 6 residents. Care is provided by aides trained in basic nursing and personal care. Board and cares are sometimes more affordable than other, higher-level care settings but are paid for privately; some allow assistance from Medicaid or the Supplemental Security Income program.
- Nursing homes, also called skilled nursing facilities, can provide both postacute and long-term care. Short-term, posthospitalization stays for skilled services (ie, physical, occupational and speech therapy, wound care, intravenous antibiotics, gastrostomy tube management) are covered by Medicare following a 3-day hospital stay. The first 20 days are covered fully and days 21 to 100 require a copay as long as there is still an ongoing skilled need. Custodial services are provided for residents who remain in the facility long term and need continued ADL assistance. These services are covered by private pay, long-term care insurance, or Medicaid.

COGNITIVE EVALUATION

The prevalence of dementia (major neurocognitive disorder) and mild cognitive impairment (minor neurocognitive disorder) increases with age. Mild dementia is often underdiagnosed without specific screening. In the busy office setting, the Mini-Cog (3-item recall and Clock Draw Test) can be used to screen for cognitive deficits in older adults with memory complaints. It can be performed by trained office staff. If the Mini-Cog returns as abnormal, further cognitive screening can be performed. Some other validated instruments for cognitive screening include the Mini Mental Status Examination, Saint Louis University Mental Status Examination, and the Montreal Cognitive

Assessment.[18] Further information on Alzheimer disease can be found elsewhere in this issue.

MOOD AND MENTAL HEALTH EVALUATION

Depression is common in older adults and adversely affects quality of life, morbidity, mortality, and health care use. Suicide rates are about twice as high in the older adult population compared with the general population, with white men more than 85 years of age at the highest risk. Many older adults with depression present to the primary care office with vague somatic complaints, such as fatigue, low energy, insomnia, or cognitive complaints. The Patient Health Questionnaire 2 (PHQ-2) (see http://www.cqaimh.org/pdf/tool_phq2.pdf) is a validated instrument used to screen for depression; it can be done quickly and can be performed by trained office staff. If abnormal, the provider should proceed with the Patient Health Questionnaire-9 (PHQ-9) to further assess depression. The PHQ-9 (see http://www.med.umich.edu/1info/FHP/practiceguides/depress/phq-9.pdf) can also be used to track response to medical therapy for depressed patients. Also, the Geriatric Depression Scale is a depression assessment tool specifically for geriatric patients, and can be acquired in multiple languages (see http://web.stanford.edu/~yesavage/GDS.html), and the Cornell Scale, which is used for depression assessment in persons with dementia (see http://geropsychiatriceducation.vch.ca/docs/edu-downloads/depression/cornell_scale_depression.pdf). These screening instruments can help identify which patients would benefit from referrals to mental health professionals, periodically assess for depression, and provide quantitative documentation of response to treatment.

PROGNOSIS AND PATIENT GOALS/ADVANCE CARE PLANNING

A follow-up concept of importance is prognosis, specifically life expectancy, if such predictors can influence the medical evaluation, management approach, and goals. Many of the decisions are guided by the patient's goals, whether it is to optimize function, prolong survival, or maximize comfort.

Advance care planning is the process by which patients and their physicians discuss the future goals of care and care preferences at the end of life. It is important to discuss these topics in a relaxed and rational environment to ensure that the decisions made reflect the type of care the individual desires. An advance directive is a legal document that comes into effect only for patients who are incapacitated and unable to speak for themselves. It allows individuals to express their wishes as well as designate a health care proxy or durable power of attorney. The older population is heterogeneous in end-of-life care preferences, and some desire comfort-oriented goals, whereas others want all treatments to prolong life regardless of condition.[19,20]

Understanding the patient's preferred goals of care may be helpful in framing treatment decisions through a shared decision-making process. Furthermore, physicians should recognize that older patients have fewer years remaining, so prognosis can be used to frame discussions about treatment options, disease prevention, and other long-term strategies. Recently many states have enacted the Medical Orders for Scope of Treatment (MOST) and Physicians Orders for Life Sustaining Treatment (POLST) forms (see http://polst.org/about/), which allow patients to have significant disease burden, in collaboration with their physicians, to document specific treatment decisions considering the patients values, alternative treatments, and goals of care, and the document becomes physicians orders. MOST and POLST forms, as well as all advance directives, should be reviewed periodically because of the changing nature of disease and functional impairment progression.

PRACTICAL APPROACH IN THE OFFICE

Clinicians understand the time constraints involved in a clinic visit and the challenges of performing a comprehensive assessment. Assessment tools and shortcuts can help reduce the burden of work in performing the initial assessment. Strategies for teamwork and cooperation with other disciplines can help make the work comprehensive but efficient. However, having an interdisciplinary assessment team is impractical in most office settings in a limited time period. Sometimes, directed and focused examinations are done when complaints can be prioritized. Also, it is wise to reevaluate

1. With whom do you live?
   Please check all that apply
   - ☐ Alone
   - ☐ Spouse or partner
   - ☐ Child
   - ☐ Other family member (specify): _____
   - ☐ Others, not family (specify): _____

2. Which of the following best describes your residence?
   - ☐ Single-family house
   - ☐ Condo
   - ☐ Apartment
   - ☐ Board & care/assisted living
   - ☐ Nursing home
   - ☐ Other (specify): _____

3. If living at a facility, please list name of person and the contact number for medical treatment orders:
   Name: _____
   Phone number: (___) _____

4. You are presently:
   - ☐ Single/never married
   - ☐ Married
   - ☐ Divorced/separated
   - ☐ Widowed
   - ☐ Living with significant other

5. How many children do you have?
   Number: _____
   Are you in regular contact with your children? ☐ Yes ☐ No

6. How much school did you complete?
   - ☐ Less than 8th grade
   - ☐ Some high school
   - ☐ High school graduate
   - ☐ Some college
   - ☐ College graduate
   - ☐ Graduate school

7. You are presently (check one):
   - ☐ Retired/not working
   - ☐ Working part-time
   - ☐ Working full-time

8. List your principal occupation and any other significant past occupations.
   1. _____
   2. _____
   3. _____
   4. _____
   5. _____

Who would you call if you were sick and needed help? (Check all that apply)
   - ☐ Spouse/partner ☐ Son ☐ Daughter ☐ Friend ☐ Neighbor
   - ☐ Other (specify): _____

A. Please list name(s) and phone number(s):
   Name: _____ Phone number: (___)
   Name: _____ Phone number: (___)
   Name: _____ Phone number: (___)

B. Do we have your permission to speak to the person(s) listed above on your behalf? ☐ Yes ☐ No

Do you employ someone to provide health related care or help you in your home? ☐ Yes ☐ No

If yes, please indicate the number of hours per day and days per week your paid helper is available to you.

Hours per day	Days per week
List number of hours:	☐ 1 ☐ 2 ☐ 3 ☐ 4 ☐ 5 ☐ 6 ☐ 7

Is this sufficient to meet your needs? ☐ Yes ☐ No

Do you get help from family members or friends in your home?
   ☐ Yes ☐ No

If yes, please indicate the number of hours per day and days per week your family member(s) or friend(s) are available to you.

Hours per day	Days per week
List number of hours:	☐ 1 ☐ 2 ☐ 3 ☐ 4 ☐ 5 ☐ 6 ☐ 7

Is this sufficient to meet your needs? ☐ Yes ☐ No

Do you provide care for a family member? ☐ Yes ☐ No

Do you drink alcohol, including beer and wine, or other alcohol (such as vodka, whiskey, gin)?
   - ☐ Daily
   - ☐ A few days a week (specify number of days: ___)
   - ☐ Less than once a week
   - ☐ Never

A. How much do you drink at a time? (One drink = 12 oz of beer or 8-9 oz of malt liquor or 5 oz of table wine or 1.5 oz of hard alcohol)
   - ☐ 1 drink
   - ☐ 2 drinks
   - ☐ 3 drinks
   - ☐ 4 drinks
   - ☐ 5 or more drinks (number: ___)

B. Has anyone ever been concerned about your drinking? ☐ Yes ☐ No

Have you ever smoked cigarettes? ☐ Yes ☐ No
If yes:
   Do you currently smoke cigarettes?
   - ☐ Yes...If yes, how many packs per day? ☐ ¼ ☐ ½ ☐ 1 ☐ 1½ ☐ 2+
   - ☐ No...If no, when did you quit? Year: _____
   For how many years did you smoke? Number of years: _____
   How many packs per day? ☐ ¼ ☐ ½ ☐ 1 ☐ 1½ ☐ 2+

Fig. 1. Previsit questionnaire: social history. (*From* Division of Geriatric Medicine. UCLA Healthcare. Pre-Visit Questionnaire. Copyright ©2016 The Regents of the University of California; with permission.)

Table 1
Previsit questionnaire: daily activities

Task	No Help Needed	Help Needed	Who Helps?
Feeding yourself			
Getting from bed to chair			
Getting to the toilet			
Getting dressed			
Bathing or showering			
Walking across the room (includes using cane or walker)			
Using the telephone			
Taking your medicines			
Preparing meals			
Managing money (like keeping track of expenses or paying bills)			
Moderately strenuous housework, such as doing the laundry			
Shopping for personal items like toiletries or medicines			
Shopping for groceries			
Driving			
Climbing a flight of stairs			
Getting to places beyond walking distance (eg, by bus, taxi, or car)			

From Division of Geriatric Medicine. UCLA Healthcare. Pre-Visit Questionnaire. Copyright ©2016 The Regents of the University of California; with permission.

certain parts of the geriatrics assessment (ie, assessing ADLs, falls, social history, mood, cognition), especially after hospitalization or major illnesses.

A previsit questionnaire can be time saving and help gather relevant information before the first visit. The questionnaire includes information about the medical history but also elaborates on elements of social history, including function, falls, incontinence, social supports, mood, vision/hearing, and advanced care planning (**Fig. 1**, **Table 1**).[21] New approaches focus on using existing office staff to help with the work flow.

With training, staff can assist with performing some assessments to save the provider time: (ie, vision and hearing, medication reconciliation, falls risk, urinary incontinence, cognitive and depression screening).

Furthermore, brief huddles before a patient session, in which the patient on the schedule is discussed, important information is alerted, and available results are provided, can facilitate a smoother work flow and maximize time efficiency.

SUMMARY

A comprehensive geriatric assessment is a multidisciplinary approach to identify medical, functional, cognitive, psychological, and socioeconomic issues in older adults. Interdisciplinary teams, consisting of the medical provider, nursing/office staff, social worker, psychologist, and others, are instrumental in developing coordinated plans of care for geriatric patients. The geriatric assessment helps determine the functional status of older adults, and can be used to determine an appropriate, safe living situation. Office staff can be trained to administer screening tools, gather data, and take on larger roles in assessing older adults to help reduce the burden of work on primary care providers.

REFERENCES

1. Boult C, Counsell S, Leipzig R, et al. The urgency of preparing primary care physicians to care for older people with chronic illness. Health Aff 2010;29(5):811–8.
2. Rosen SL, Reuben DB. Geriatric assessment tools. Mt Sinai J Med 2011;78:489.
3. Inouye S, Studenski S, Tinetti ME, et al. Geriatric syndromes: clinical, research and policy implications of a core geriatric concept. J Am Geriatr Soc 2007; 55(5):780–91.
4. Kass MA, Heuer DK, Higginbotham EJ, et al. The Ocular Hypertension Treatment Study: a randomized trial determines that topical ocular hypotensive medication delays or prevents the onset of primary open-angle glaucoma. Arch Ophthalmol 2002;120(6):701–13.
5. US Preventive Services Task Force. The guide to clinical preventive services 2014. Agency for Health Care Research and Quality; 2012.
6. Roberts RO, Jacobsen SJ, Rhodes T, et al. Urinary incontinence in a community-based cohort: prevalence and health-care seeking. J Am Geriatr Soc 1998;46(4): 467–72.
7. Laimer M, Kramer-Reinstadler K, Rauchenzauner M, et al. Effect of mirtazapine treatment on body composition and metabolism. J Clin Psychiatry 2006;67: 421–4.
8. Bloom HG, Ahmed I, Alessi CA, et al. Evidence-based recommendations for the assessment and management of sleep disorders in older persons. J Am Geriatr Soc 2009;57(5):761–89.
9. Alessi CA, Martin JL, Webber AP, et al. Randomized, controlled trial of a nonpharmacologic intervention to improve abnormal sleep/wake patterns in nursing home residents. J Am Geriatr Soc 2005;53(5):803–10.
10. Carney CE, Buysse DJ, Ancoli-Israel S, et al. The consensus sleep diary: standardizing prospective sleep self-monitoring. Sleep 2012;35(2):287–302.
11. Schroeck J, Ford J, Conway E, et al. Review of safety and efficacy of sleep medicines in older adults. Clin Ther 2016;38:2340–72.
12. Gill TM, Robison JT, Tinetti ME. Difficulty and dependence: two components of the disability continuum among community-living older persons. Ann Intern Med 1998;128:96.
13. Inouye SK, Peduzzi PN, Robison JT, et al. Importance of functional measures in predicting mortality among older hospitalized patients. JAMA 1998;279:1187.
14. Reuben DB, Solomon DH. Assessment in geriatrics. Of caveats and names. J Am Geriatr Soc 1989;37:570.
15. Tinetti ME, Williams CS. Falls, injuries due to falls, and the risk of admission to a nursing home. N Engl J Med 1997;337(18):1279–84.
16. Okumiya K, Matsubayashi K, Nakamura T, et al. The timed "up & go" test is a useful predictor of falls in community-swelling older people. J Am Geriatr Soc 1998; 46(7):928–30.
17. National Institute of Justice. Available at: https://www.nij.gov/topics/crime/elder-abuse/pages/welcome.aspx. Accessed April 27, 2017.

18. Lin JS, O'Connor E, Rossom RC, et al. Screening for cognitive impairment in older adults: a systematic review for the U.S. Preventative Services Task Force. Ann Intern Med 2013;159(9):601–12.
19. Keeler E, Guralnik JM, Tian H, et al. The impact of functional status on life expectancy in older persons. J Gerontol A Biol Sci Med Sci 2010;65:727.
20. Reuben DB, Tinetti ME. Goal-oriented patient care–an alternative health outcomes paradigm. N Engl J Med 2012;366:777.
21. Reuben DB, Leonard SD. Office-based assessment of the older adult. UptoDate; 2016. Available at: http://www.uptodate.com/contents/office-based-assessment-of-the-older-adult.

Managing Polypharmacy in the 15-Minute Office Visit

Demetra Antimisiaris, PharmD, BCGP, FASCP[a,b,c],*, Timothy Cutler, PharmD, BCGP[d]

KEYWORDS

- Polypharmacy • Medication reconciliation • Potentially inappropriate medications
- Beers criteria • Morisky scale • Geriatric syndromes
- Comprehensive medication management • Drug interactions

KEY POINTS

- The prevalence of polypharmacy is significant and growing, with the United States leading the world in medication per capita use. Older adults live with polypharmacy due to high chronic and acute disease burden.
- Polypharmacy (medication management) skills are essential when caring for older adults and can offer improved quality measure outcomes and improved reimbursements.
- The health care system and multiple providers contribute to the syndrome of polypharmacy. At minimum, a thorough medication reconciliation and medication management session should be performed at least annually.
- Proactive implementation of a systematic polypharmacy management program (despite the 15-minute office visit rush) is preferable to reactive management of sometimes serious medication-related problems.
- Efficient involvement of the patient, the office team, and community resources can result in improved medication management and outcomes.

INTRODUCTION

The American Board of Internal Medicine Foundation launched an initiative called Choosing Wisely, with the goal of advancing dialogue on wasteful or unnecessary medical tests, treatments, and procedures (American Medical Board Foundation. Choosing Wisely. Available at http://www.choosingwisely.org). The Choosing

The authors have nothing to disclosures.
[a] Pharmacy and Medication Management Program, Department of Pharmacology and Toxicology, University of Louisville, 501 East Broadway, Suite 240, Louisville, KY 40202, USA; [b] Department of Neurology, University of Louisville, 501 East Broadway, Suite 240, Louisville, KY 40202, USA; [c] Department of Family Medicine and Geriatrics, University of Louisville, 501 East Broadway, Suite 240, Louisville, KY 40202, USA; [d] Department of Clinical Pharmacy, UCSF School of Pharmacy, 533 Parnassus Avenue U585, UCSF POBox 0622, San Francisco, CA 94117, USA
* Corresponding author. Department of Family Medicine and Geriatrics, University of Louisville, 501 East Broadway, Suite 240, Louisville, KY 40202.
E-mail address: demetra.antimisiaris@louisville.edu

Prim Care Clin Office Pract 44 (2017) 413–428
http://dx.doi.org/10.1016/j.pop.2017.04.003
0095-4543/17/© 2017 Elsevier Inc. All rights reserved.

Wisely campaign asked national organizations representing medical specialists to identify areas of potential waste and the American Geriatrics Society in 2013 released their Choosing Wisely list of 10 things clinicians and patients should question; 7 of the 10 Choosing Wisely recommendations pertain to medication use.[1]

The need for the care of older adults has increased over the past several years, especially as it relates to the use of medications in older adults. From the years 1998 to 2008, the overall rate of office visits for those over age 65 increased by 13%. For those visits where medications were prescribed or continued, patients over age 65 had the highest increase in visits (31%) compared with any other age group.[2] In the new era of quality measure reporting and incentives, management of medications in the elderly has become an important element of primary care. For example, the Physician Quality Reporting System and the Medicare Access and CHIP Reauthorization Act implemented by the Centers for Medicare and Medicaid Services list several measures that evaluate appropriate medication management as an integral part of outcomes ranging from management of neuropsychiatric symptoms of dementia, plan of care for falls, urinary incontinence plan of care, diabetes control, statin therapy for prevention of cardiovascular disease, and medication reconciliation postdischarge. Failure to achieve quality thresholds results in lower Medicare payments to individual and group practices.

Any symptom in an elderly patient should be considered a medication related problem until proved otherwise
—Gurwitz J, Monane M, Monane S, and Avorn J. Brown University Long-Term Care Quality Letter, 2001.[3]

The challenges of appropriate management of medications in older adults can be broken down into the following areas: multimorbidity, polypharmacy PIMs in the elderly, underuse of medications, and adherence and access to medications. There are several challenges specific to primary care providers (PCPs) when managing these issues in older adults, which include the brevity of the typical office visit; medically complex patients; multiple specialists who contribute to a patient's overall polypharmacy; frequent hospitalizations and transitions of care; lack of high-quality evidence to guide prescribing for older adults, in particular the old-old, who are typically over 80 years of age; and the fact that evidence-based guidelines rely on clinical trials that typically exclude multimorbid and frail older adults.[4–7]

Polypharmacy is traditionally defined in the literature as the use of 5 or more chronic medications, the use of inappropriate medications, or medications that are not clinically warranted.[8] Historically, the 15-minute office visit consists of approximately 7 minutes dedicated to establishment of the problem, 3.5 minutes to work on the problem, and 3.5 minutes dedicated to medications.[4] Patients living with polypharmacy do not have much opportunity to have their overall medication needs addressed in a clinic visit. In the era of quality measure reimbursement, these challenges also present an opportunity to demonstrate improvement of outcomes and leveraging quality-based reimbursements through proactive attention to management of polypharmacy.

There is increasing evidence of the value, decreased morbidity, and mortality as well as return on investment when focused medication management occurs.[9–15] The intent of this article is to provide some strategies PCPs to provide overall polypharmacy management for the increasing cohort of older adult patients expected in the coming years.

ACHIEVING OPTIMAL POLYPHARMACY MANAGEMENT IN THE OLDER ADULT
Focus on Monitoring Medication Use

Older adults live with multiple chronic conditions, underlying incidents of acute medical and functional problems, which leads to multiple transitions of care. Multimorbidity and transitions of care leads to polypharmacy, which is considered a geriatric syndrome. Geriatric syndromes are problems that are highly prevalent in older adults, especially frail older adults. Geriatric syndromes do not refer to an organic disease but multifactorial issues involved with multiple problems, leading to added impairment and negative impact on quality of life. Examples of geriatric syndromes include but are not limited to dizziness, cognitive impairment, delirium, falls, frailty, syncope, urinary incontinence, and polypharmacy. A core principle of the management of polypharmacy in older adults is avoidance of PIMS. Ultimately, determination of whether a medication is inappropriate or not is highly individualized and often circumstantial as well. A medication that is inappropriate now, for example highly elevated carbidopa-levodopa doses in a patient long term on high doses, may become appropriate again after a carbidopa-levodopa high-dose holiday. Medications that are considered potentially inappropriate in general can be found in 2 established resources that serve as guidance on PIMS in older adults. These 2 resources are the Beers criteria and the START and STOPP criteria.[16,17] The use of the Beers criteria and START and STOPP criteria is discussed later.

Polypharmacy and the health care system: the care of older adults is typically provided by multiple specialists, in addition to PCPs, as well as several ancillary care providers. A silo effect can occur, where each care provider works on a specific problem without ever having an opportunity to communicate or discuss with the other providers. Adding to the silo effect are the various care settings that older adults frequent, such as hospitals, assisted living residences, nursing homes, postdischarge rehabilitation facilities, adult day care, and more. The complexity and velocity of care changes multimorbid older adults live with lead to a dearth of opportunities to perform needed comprehensive medication reconciliation (CMR), leading to unchecked polypharmacy and undesirable outcomes.[18] Each transition of care should warrant a CMR, and even when a CMR is just performed at least annually, up to 90% of patients have some form of medication-related problem identified.[19] CMR and comprehensive medication management (CMM) are challenging to fit into a busy primary care (or specialty) office practice. Medicare offers an annual CMM for beneficiaries through Medicare D. Medication therapy management service is provided through a Medicare patient's pharmacy benefits manager and patients can be referred for a CMM by helping them to contact their pharmacy benefits manager and be assigned a consultant. There are innovative models, particularly associated with patient-centered medical home models, which provide the operationalization methods (billing models) to provide improved CMR and CMM in the office practice.[20,21]

One immediate means of implementing improved medication management is to focus on monitoring and pharmacovigilance. There is evidence that medication monitoring is an often-missed opportunity to prevent adverse drug events (ADEs).[22] The major factors leading to ADEs in ambulatory community-dwelling older adults have been identified as rooted in problems with monitoring, prescribing, and adherence. Monitoring is involved in approximately 60% of ADEs, prescribing involved in 58%, and adherence involved in 60% (more than 1 of these factors could contribute to each incident).[22]

Two major studies of older adults evaluating emergency department visits and hospitalizations for ADEs found that drugs, such as digoxin, warfarin, insulins, oral antiplatelet agents, and oral hypoglycemic agents, were responsible for a majority of hospitalizations (39% and 67%, respectively) and PIMs included on the Beers list were responsible for only 1.2% of hospitalizations. Digoxin, warfarin, insulins, oral antiplatelets, and oral hypoglycemic medications were 35 times more likely to result in hospitalization than medications considered potentially inappropriate for older adults.[23,24] Although the Beers list of PIMs in the elderly is important, the medications consistently found to result in older adults' hospital visits are medications that are commonly in use, the monitoring parameters of which are well known. These studies support the idea that potentially missed monitoring of routine, daily use medications, for chronic disease can result in serious medication misadventure in the elderly. Additional evidence supporting the need for appropriate medication monitoring includes a systematic review, which evaluates preventable ADEs in ambulatory care patients, and found that 45% of preventable adverse drug reactions were due to inadequate monitoring and 16% due to ignoring or missing a clinical or laboratory result.[25]

Because the effort required to have an impact on patient adherence is labor intensive and challenging, PCPs working toward more effective medication monitoring may be more easily achieved than working on adherence[26] (CMM consults through Medicare D can provide a means of working on adherence as well as peer disease support groups and midlevel providers). Monitoring medication use in the office practice is achievable when a systematic approach is implemented, such as that used to monitor international normalization ratio for persons receiving warfarin.

Appropriate monitoring of medication use requires setting up a system to provide periodic interval monitoring for each medication a patient is using. Such a system might include assigning tracking of monitoring to medical staff, because sometimes complex medication use tracks 20 or more medications for 1 patient. Similar systems are often used for international normalization ratio tracking in patients using warfarin. Alternately, electronic records could be designed to track missed monitoring. Besides tracking intervals of monitoring for each medication, a clinic team could perform other tasks, such as database scanning for recommended monitoring appropriate for each drug and drug interaction evaluation. Clerkship students, midlevel providers, or other members of the primary care team can perform this routine work as well.

People often think of drug monitoring as making sure the laboratory monitoring associated with a drug is completed. But other important forms of monitoring include following drug monograph recommendations to track and document common adverse events for each medication, common medication–disease adverse events, drug-drug interactions, and monitoring renal, hepatic, and cytochrome enzyme clearance interactions.

Lastly, a commonly overlooked form of monitoring is monitoring for efficacy. If efficacy is nonexistent, then a medication should be discontinued from use (**Box 1**).

Algorithms and processes for monitoring appropriateness and need of medication use in older adults have been created and can be useful in developing a systematic approach to medication use monitoring[27,28] (see algorithm by Garfinkle and colleagues, referenced in *UptoDate*).[29]

Heightened efforts to monitor drug use would work toward decreasing the incidence of overlooked pharmacovigilance, thus preventing emergency department visits and hospitalizations.[30,31]

Deprescribing and Prescribing of Omitted Therapies

Deprescribing has been demonstrated as a useful tool in optimization of functional status and diminishing medication-related problem risks, where the number of medications taken by a patient is the single most important predictor of inappropriate

---

Box 1
Medication monitoring check list

- Efficacy—if not efficacious, consider deprescribing.

- Laboratory monitoring—track, follow-up, and implement at appropriate intervals.

- Drug-drug interactions—run a drug interaction checker periodically and document presence or absence of drug interactions.

- Drug-disease interactions

- Monitor renal, hepatic clearance.

- Keep aware of cytochrome enzyme clearance interactions—for example, a course of fluconazole can cause phenytoin to become toxic.

---

medication use.[32] Deprescribing is the process of stopping or tapering medications to minimize inappropriate medication use or polypharmacy. The goal is to target one at a time and to avoid changing too many items at once or abruptly.

Consideration of deprescribing of a medication: look for medications that have no valid reason for being used; evaluate the overall risk of drug-induced harm; assess current or future benefit versus risk; prioritize discontinuation and consider removal of medications with lowest benefit to heightened harm risk first; and implement a plan to discontinue (perhaps a taper) and monitor follow-up. Typically, the medications that have no accompanying diagnosis, problems, or obvious reason for use are there because they are treating underappreciated side effects of other medications. It is best to strive to manage the side effects of offending agents first by optimizing dose or selection of another medication for the problem rather than making the drug tolerable by treating the side effect.

Scan for PIMs for elderly patients by consulting criteria regarding PIM and appropriate medication use in older adults, such as the Beers criteria and START and STOPP criteria. These criteria also present evidence and expert opinion regarding underprescribed medications that should be used in the elderly (ie, warfarin in atrial fibrillation patients who fall; although is counterintuitive, the supporting evidence is presented).[16,17]

Avoid the Prescribing Cascade

Systematic medication monitoring should accompany vigilance in avoiding the prescribing cascade. The prescribing cascade occurs when a medication is used to treat the side effect of another medication (**Fig. 1**). For most cases, the prescribing cascade dynamic is undesirable but sometimes it is intentional. Examples of prescribing a medication to treat the side effects of another medication are (1) a patient taking antipsychotic agents resulting in extrapyramidal symptoms, and anticholinergic agents are prescribed to treat the extrapyramidal symptoms when the benefit of antipsychotic agent use outweighs the risks, and (2) the use of a stimulant laxative for patients receiving chronic opioids.

Individualization of Medication Use

An important consideration in the care of older adults is the need for individualization of care due to the heterogeneous health status of persons aged 65 and older. Most single-disease practice guidelines do not include evidence derived from multimorbidity patients or persons with advanced age.[33] With age, patients become

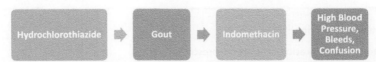

Fig. 1. Prescribing CASCADE-In this example, hydrochlorothiazide used for hypertension, eventually leads to gout, which is treated with indomethacin, which becomes the cause of dangerously high blood pressure, nose bleeds, and confusion (not recommended for older adults per Beers criteria, yet a drug of choice for gout treatment). The prescribing CASCADE described here is a real case, resolved permanently by substitution of hydrochlorothiazide with low dose amlodipine.

physiologically and functionally very different from one another due to chronic disease and individual morbidity burdens, which leads to individualized life expectancies and physiologic reserve. The physiologic changes that occur with age, such as diminished renal function and increased percent body fat with decreased percent body water, have an impact on the way medications perform pharmacokinetically, and altered pharmacodynamic response is influenced by these pharmacokinetic changes as well as underlying physiologic pathologies, such as impaired baroreceptor response. Age is only a surrogate marker for many of the factors to consider in choosing treatment options. There are people in their early 60s with serious debility and others near 90 who are busy climbing mountains. The Food and Drug Administration (FDA) recently mandated increased inclusion of more subjects over 65 years of age in clinical trials, yet most trials do not reflect the actual proportion of older adults living with the disease for which the medication is being tested.[34] The effects of comorbidities on disease-specific outcomes are inadequately studied in chronic disease trials from which clinical guidelines are derived.[35,36]

The cornerstone of treatment recommendations are chronic disease guidelines and other disease-specific guidelines resulting in the use multiple medications, especially in those with multiple conditions. The ability to sustain high drug burden and other interventions is relative to factors, such as frailty, physiologic reserve, and total disease burden.[37–39] Conversely, there is the question of the impact of medications on functional status.[40] Polypharmacy resulting from multiple providers following disease practice guidelines, resulting in untested combinations of medications, can be associated with suboptimal functional status and negative outcomes.[41–44] That said, robust older adults who are living with minimal chronic disease burden and minimal functional impairment can benefit from long-term disease prevention just as a younger person can.

Application of clinical practice guidelines to the older adult patient requires special assessment and consideration: Are patients robust or frail? What is their functional status? Is the current functional status temporary or long term? How heavy is their comorbidity and geriatric syndrome burden? What are their preferences and goals of care? How does a patient's quality of life interplay with these considerations? Is the patient able to adhere to treatment? What are the risks versus benefits of treatment? What is the time horizon to benefit versus patient's life expectancy?

Consider the recent changes in the United States guidelines for diabetes, lipids, and hypertension. All of them have added a statement of individualization of care for those over 80 years of age, and the statin use guidelines have explicitly included consideration of 10-year cardiovascular risk in determining medication use choices.[45–47] These major chronic disease guidelines have acknowledged that application of the evidence, such as time to benefit, time to harm, and other parameters, are applied differently to individuals outside the (younger and less medically complex) study population, such as some older adults.

The American Geriatrics Society Expert Panel on the Care of Older Adults with Multi-morbidity[48] recommends a stepwise approach. The approach explains an algorithm that includes patient's primary concern, consideration of relevant evidence, prognosis, interactions with and among treatments and conditions, benefits versus harms, communication, and reassessment for alignment with preferences, feasibility, adherence, and benefit at selected intervals. For some patients, careful consideration of multimorbidity effects on treatments can have a marked impact on medication management decisions. In addition to the American Geriatrics Society approach, a classic algorithm to help determine appropriateness of medication use is the Medication Appropriateness Index, illustrated in **Box 2**.

Lastly, after ensuring a patient's understanding of conditions, medications, and risks versus benefits, the importance of finding out if the patient wants to take the medications being prescribed or recommended to take should not be overlooked. For a comprehensive online review of person-centered medication use optimization, refer to the British National Institute for Health and Care Excellence guideline.[49]

As for medication dosing, the rule of thumb in terms of titrating medication dose is "start low and go slow." Although medications typically are accompanied by target dosing, for the frail elderly, targeting the minimum effective dose is a safer approach.

Verification of appropriate renal dose adjustment should be checked for each medication an older adult patient is taking. The renal dose adjustment should be made using the Cockroft-Gault equation for estimated creatinine clearance for 2 reasons: first, the Cockroft-Gault method is the FDA standard by which dose recommendations in the drug monographs are reported (thus to use another equation would be like comparing apples to oranges), and second, the Cockroft-Gault equation underestimates renal clearance compared with the estimated glomerular filtration rate, Modificaiton of Diet in Renal Disease, or gold standard of 24-hour urine collection. Underestimation of renal function is typically safer for older adults regarding renal dose adjustment for medications. The Cockroft-Gault equation is easily found in point-of-care applications, such as Epocrates, Lexicomp, and online support sites, such as GlobalRPh or National Kidney Foundation. Typically, height, weight, and

---

Box 2
Medication appropriateness index

1. Is there an indication for the drug?

2. Is the medication effective for the condition?

3. Is the dosage correct?

4. Are the directions correct?

5. Are the directions practical?

6. Are there clinically significant drug-drug interactions?

7. Are there clinically significant drug-disease/condition interactions?

8. Is there unnecessary duplication with other drugs?

9. Is the duration of therapy acceptable?

10. Is this drug the least expensive alternative compared with others of equal usefulness?

From Hanlon JT, Schmader KE, Samsa GP, et al. A method for assessing drug therapy appropriateness. J Clin Epidemiol 1992;45(10):1045–51; with permission.

serum creatinine level are needed at hand to use these calculators. If there is not a serum creatinine level, for persons over 65 year of age, a minimum creatinine clearance can be estimated using serum creatinine = 1 mg/dL. In persons over 65, even if the serum creatinine is less than 1 mg/dL, clinical medication consultants typically round up to 1 mg/dL because most persons over 65 have some degree of sarcopenia, which can cause misleading creatinine levels for estimating renal clearance. Also, it is important to use stable serum creatinine levels. Much like blood pressure, one reading may reflect a transient condition due to medication use, dehydration, or some other renal accident.[50]

IMPLEMENTATION OF POLYPHARMACY MANAGEMENT IN THE 15-MINUTE OFFICE VISIT

It is important to recognize that optimal polypharmacy management does not occur in 15 minutes. Proactively and systematically, however, checking off some of the elements of optimal polypharmacy management during each visit and repeating periodically (annually perhaps) is preferable to addressing polypharmacy when problems arise (**Fig. 2**).

Medication Reconciliation

Medication reconciliation is typically defined as getting the most accurate list of medications a patient is using. Appropriate medication reconciliation involves patient and caregiver interviews, lists from health records, pharmacy records, hospitalization

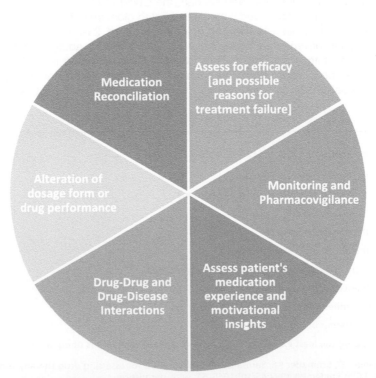

Fig. 2. Proposed checklist of polypharmacy management checklist items.

records, controlled substance refill reporting, and accounting for over-the-counter medication, supplements, herbal products, and vitamins. The process of getting accurate data is impacted by transitions of care, a patient's ability to report and keep records, clinical team time, and resources. Much of the work of medication reconciliation can be given to midlevel providers, office staff, student volunteers working in a clinic, and health care professional trainees. The data-gathering aspect can be done as much as possible before the 15-minute office visit with system implementation of medication reconciliation protocol.

The brown bag assessment means that patients bring everything they are taking at the current time in a bag to each appointment. The brown bag assessment is the gold standard for medication reconciliation (if patients remember to bring everything they are taking). The ideal is to go through the brown bag assessment at each office visit, although once per year at minimum is helpful. Sometimes patients omit some products they are taking because they do not assume, for example, that an over-the-counter medication should be part of a brown bag assessment; perhaps they perceive the brown bag should be only prescription medications. Therefore, it is important to provide a bit of training for patients to ensure that they understand they are to bring everything. Patients should also bring a list of medications they take, if they keep one, for comparison.

Medication reconciliation and initial medication use interviewing can be done by office staff, medical assistants, volunteer students, or trainees before a 15-minute office visit by going through the process of listing the contents of the bag. It is important to train whoever does the brown bag assessment to ask open-ended questions to find out if there is anything missing. Open-ended questions about how a patient is taking each medication should be recorded and compared with the instructions on the labels.

Staff or volunteers can also work to gather medication data for patients ahead of an office visit by requesting hospital discharge records, pharmacy records, and controlled substance reporting records to save time and to help ensure complete medication reconciliation during the office visit. Health Insurance Portability and Accountability Act training and credentialing for patient interaction and care are requirements before enlisting staff or volunteers to help with brown bag assessments and medication reconciliation data collection. Regarding the added time required to provide for older adult patients in the clinic setting in general, precepting students can be a bidirectionally beneficial activity. Students learn much about the complexity of patient care and gain experience, and they can be helpful to a practice setting.

Monitoring and Pharmacovigilance

- For each prescription and over-the-counter medication, consult point-of-care drug databases or the FDA drug monograph prescribing information to document, for each medication, routine laboratory studies, renal dose adjustments, top side effects, and drug-disease interactions.
- For herbal products and supplements, consult the NIH Complementary and Alternative Medicine Herbal and Natural Products Web site, where there is a list of databases that can offer resources for monitoring these products (see section on herbal products and supplements). Typically, drug interaction checkers, when including herbal, supplements, and vitamins, flag problems of product-disease or product-drug interactions accurately.

When a patient is using drugs that are new to market, a heightened approach to monitoring should be adapted. As discussed previously, clinical studies tend to exclude older adult patients, in particular frail and multimorbid patients. The exclusion of the very old and frail from safety and efficacy trials that bring drugs to market, means, expected monitoring and adverse effect recommendations for frail older adults is uncertain in new to market drugs. The case of Vioxx® (Rofecoxib) is an example of a new-to-market drug that possessed a high risk of ADEs, which was discovered through post-marketing surveillance, and a serious threat to older adults. Older adults are more susceptible to unexpected adverse outcomes with new-to-market drugs due to lack of physiologic reserve and lack of data that from postmarketing surveillance.[51]

Clinical Pearl

New-to-market medications should be avoided in older adults; older adults tend to be excluded from new drug trials, and postmarketing data typically reveal problems with medications in older adults.

Drug-Drug Interactions

At minimum, running a patient's prescription and over-the-counter medications, herbal products, and supplements through an interaction checker should be done periodically.[52] There are several available in point-of-care applications, such as Epocrates or Lexicomp, or online. Patients can be advised to help perform their own polypharmacy pharmacovigilance by running their lists through interaction checkers online, such as those found at Drugs.com or RxList. The results can then be reviewed with patients to improve self-management and medication use literacy. The patient or clinic staff could have the process of running a drug interaction checker done before the appointment with the provider. The frequency for performing interaction checkers is dependent on patients and the consistency of their total medication and product use.

Assess for Medication and Over-the-Counter Herbal or Supplement Product Efficacy

One important and commonly overlooked aspect of polypharmacy management is assessment of medication efficacy. Some medications are difficult to assess for efficacy because their effectiveness is targeted at long-term prevention, and a person's life expectancy is a variable which, therefore impacts the definition of efficacy. But, in frail older adults, when medications are used to treat a problem that affects quality of life or end-stage disease, assessment of efficacy is not as difficult to determine. One means of assessment of medication efficacy in patients treated for end-stage disease symptoms or symptoms affecting quality of life is to withhold the medication if safe to do so for a short interval to assess utility and safety of that medication's use. Two examples where discovering ineffective medication is useful in older adults are overactive bladder medications and loop diuretics used for lower extremity edema in patients with venous stasis. Both medication classes present significant risk for the frail and older patients who use them.

Overactive bladder medications can cause cognitive impairment and cardiac events as well as occasionally inducing overflow incontinence by causing increased postvoid residual. Patients often fail treatment in part because other modes of treatment besides pharmacotherapy should be used simultaneously, such as routine toileting. The etiologies are so complex that medications alone are not always the solution.[53,54] A study of 103,250 patients with mean age of 58.7 over 24 months taking medications for overactive bladder found that time to treatment failure was 159 days, with 91.7% failing to meet treatment goals.[55]

Lower extremity edema is common because of inactivity and diminished homeostatic venous capacity, and, in some cases, the chronic use of loop diuretics achieves little improvement while placing patients at increased risk of electrolyte disorders, impaired renal function, and stimulation of the renin angiotensin system and volume depletion.[56] Often, lack of further evaluation to determine the correct etiology leads to inappropriate loop diuretic use long-term without efficacy.[57,58] For those cases of loop diuretics resulting in little efficacy, management with increased movement and extremity elevation has been can be an effective alternative.

In general, aggressively applying a single pharmacologic mode can result in inefficacy in older patients because the problems older patients experience is so often multifactorial. One reason for treatment failure and inefficacy is that the multifactorial aspects to geriatric syndromes and problems are not evaluated. There are some medications that have not been shown widely effective, such as treatments for Alzheimer dementia, yet are difficult to stop because the decision about efficacy involves the beliefs of the caregivers and subjective findings.[59] Herbals, supplements, and vitamins are other examples of a category for which it is not easy to prove efficacy yet difficult to get patients to give up because of their belief and expectations. With herbals, supplements, and vitamins, the risk of unknown effects is problematic and it is worth attempting to gain patient trust to stop them if not needed. Explaining that herbals, supplements, and vitamins are not regulated as prescription and over-the-counter medications are by the FDA sometimes helps Improve patient awareness.

Assess Alteration of Dosage Forms and the Impact of Food or Acid Suppression Therapy

Any patient, especially a person with swallowing difficulties, is liable to split tablets or open or crush capsules just to be able to take them. The challenge is that the practice of dosage form alteration can significantly alter the way the medications perform and lead to significant toxicity.[60] An Australian study showed that 17% of medications altered before administration had potential to cause increased toxicity, decreased efficacy, and safety or stability concerns, and the incidence of drug dosage form alteration was 46% in the high care setting, 34% in the intermediate care setting, and 2% in the low care setting.[61] Therefore, an important component of polypharmacy management is at least occasionally (perhaps once annually) asking patients if they split or crush any tablets that they are taking. These data might help identify any treatment failures, toxicities, or adverse effects.

If medication treatment failures or abnormalities are observed, assessment of the potential impact of acid suppression therapy and bariatric surgery should be considered.[62–64] Recently geriatrics practice are starting to see the first cohort of aging Roux-en-Y gastric bypass patients. They may present with nutrient deficiencies, which appear at first to be cognitive impairment of Alzheimer or other type of dementia, or sometimes with inability to get relief from pain medications as well as treatment failures. Also, it should be considered that when medications are developed, they are designed to perform under normal gastric circumstances in which the gastric pH is approximately 1.0, and chronic proton pump inhibitor use can elevate the gastric pH to over 4, which can alter the performance of some medications.[62,65,66]

The effect of combining medications with food should be evaluated for evaluation of medication efficacy and possible link to side effects, such as upset stomach and nausea. With tamsulosin [Flomax], the recommendations are to take one-half hour after the same meal each day and to not crush or chew. The presence of food, however, causes a lower plasma peak and lower bioavailability than an empty stomach (30% increase in bioavailability and up to 70% higher plasma peak), meaning that instead of increasing the dose of tamsulosin from 0.4 mg to 0.8 mg, a provider might try having the patient take it on an empty stomach in the morning, one-half hour before breakfast, to attempt to gain better efficacy, if the patient can tolerate the drug on an empty stomach.

Assess Patient Medication Use Experience and Patient-centered Medication Use Risks

There are multiple patient-centered factors that influence successful medication use and risk of medication use failures, for example, health literacy, cognitive impairment, recent transitions of care (hospitalization and rehabilitation stay), socioeconomic barriers to consistent medication access, and multiple providers. The following checklist represents patient-centered screens for medication or polypharmacy related patient-centered risks:

- Health literacy screening[67]
- Morisky scale (adherence screen)[68]
- Any recent hospitalization or transitions of care or institutionalization?
- Barrier to medication access
  - Transportation
  - Medicare D doughnut hole
  - Uncovered medications

Motivational interviewing to detect a patient's actual medication experience includes the use of open-ended questions. Ideally, going through the medication list one by one and asking what the medication is for, is it working, and if there are there any problems can be revealing. The ultimate driver of adherence is the belief that a medication works, which is strongly supported by feedback either by perceivable action or fostered by health care professional education and health literacy enforcement. Thus, medications, such as zolpidem (Ambien), which provide immediate feedback that they work, are adhered to closely. For statins, adherence is not driven as much by feedback. The discovery of subtle problems related to a patient's medication experience or common barriers, such as uncovered medications, might trigger a good time for a referral for CMM services (through Medicare D benefit or other, as discussed previously).

SUMMARY

The management of polypharmacy in a 15-minute office visit presents a significant challenge in older adults, yet the PCP and the patient-centered medical home seem to be the optimal places to implement overall medication management. Creating a systematic method to address polypharmacy in older patients, by looking to minimize the use of PIMs, performing CMR at least once annually (perhaps as part of the Medicare annual wellness visit), working with the office or extended community team (referral for CMM through Medicare D partners), and ensuring appropriate monitoring can go a long way toward improving outcomes and avoiding medication-related misadventure. Each practice has different polypharmacy management needs based on patient demographics, location, and health system parameters. Fortunately, there are growing varieties of resources online and in communities to make successful medication management a reality. Taking the time to curate a system and network for a practice will provide significant returns on investment via avoided hospitalization, increased billing levels, and heightened quality measure bonuses, but most of all, patients will feel empowered and more functional with improved medication management and avoidance of unnecessary polypharmacy.

REFERENCES

1. McCormick WC. Revised AGS Choosing Wisely((R)) list: changes to help guide older adult care conversations. J Gerontol Nurs 2015;41(5):49–50.
2. Cherry DLC, Decker SL. Population aging and the use of office-based physician services. NCHS data brief, no 41. Hyattsville (MD): National Center for Health Statistics; 2010. CDC websight.
3. Gurwitz J, Monane M, Monane S, et al. Brown University long-term care quality letter. American Society on Aging—National Council on Aging Annual Conference. 2001.
4. Van Spall HG, Toren A, Kiss A, et al. Eligibility criteria of randomized controlled trials published in high-impact general medical journals: a systematic sampling review. JAMA 2007;297(11):1233–40.
5. Tai-Seale M, McGuire T. Time is up: increasing shadow price of time in primary-care office visits. Health Econ 2012;21(4):457–76.
6. Sganga F, Landi F, Ruggiero C, et al. Polypharmacy and health outcomes among older adults discharged from hospital: results from the CRIME study. Geriatr Gerontol Int 2015;15(2):141–6.
7. Gamble JM, Hall JJ, Marrie TJ, et al. Medication transitions and polypharmacy in older adults following acute care. Ther Clin Risk Manag 2014;10:189–96.
8. Fried TR, O'Leary J, Towle V, et al. Health outcomes associated with polypharmacy in community-dwelling older adults: a systematic review. J Am Geriatr Soc 2014;62(12):2261–72.
9. Garfinkel D, Zur-Gil S, Ben-Israel J. The war against polypharmacy: a new cost-effective geriatric-palliative approach for improving drug therapy in disabled elderly people. Isr Med Assoc J 2007;9(6):430–4.
10. Hilmer SN, Mager DE, Simonsick EM, et al. A drug burden index to define the functional burden of medications in older people. Arch Intern Med 2007;167(8):781–7.
11. Hilmer SN, Gnjidic D, Abernethy DR. Drug Burden Index for international assessment of the functional burden of medications in older people. J Am Geriatr Soc 2014;62(4):791–2.
12. Jodar-Sanchez F, Malet-Larrea A, Martin JJ, et al. Cost-utility analysis of a medication review with follow-up service for older adults with polypharmacy in community pharmacies in Spain: the conSIGUE program. Pharmacoeconomics 2015;33(6):599–610.
13. Wittayanukorn S, Westrick SC, Hansen RA, et al. Evaluation of medication therapy management services for patients with cardiovascular disease in a self-insured employer health plan. J Manag Care Pharm 2013;19(5):385–95.
14. Brummel A, Lustig A, Westrich K, et al. Best practices: improving patient outcomes and costs in an ACO through comprehensive medication therapy management. J Manag Care Spec Pharm 2014;20(12):1152–8.
15. Gazda NP, Berenbrok LA, Ferreri SP. Comparison of two Medication Therapy Management Practice Models on Return on Investment. J Pharm Pract 2016;30(3):282–5.
16. By the American Geriatrics Society Beers Criteria Update Expert Panel. American Geriatrics Society 2015 updated beers criteria for potentially inappropriate medication use in older adults. J Am Geriatr Soc 2015;63(11):2227–46.
17. O'Mahony D, O'Sullivan D, Byrne S, et al. STOPP/START criteria for potentially inappropriate prescribing in older people: version 2. Age Ageing 2015;44(2):213–8.

18. Cipolle RJ, Cipolle RJ, Morley PC, et al. Pharmaceutical care practice. 3rd edition. New York: McGraw-Hill; 2012.
19. Woodall T, Landis SE, Galvin SL, et al. Provision of annual wellness visits with comprehensive medication management by a clinical pharmacist practitioner. Am J Health Syst Pharm 2017;74(4):218–23.
20. Collaborative PCPC. Integrating comprehensive medicaiton management to optimize patient outcomes. 2nd edition. PCPCC Resource Guide on Integrating CMM. Washington, DC: Patient Centered Primacy Care Collaborative; 2012. Available at: https://www.pcpcc.org/sites/default/files/media/medmanagement.pdf. Accessed February 1, 2017.
21. American College of Clinical Pharmacists. Comprehensive medication management in team-based care. Washington, DC: American College of Clinical Pharmacists Brief; 2016.
22. Gurwitz JH, Field TS, Harrold LR, et al. Incidence and preventability of adverse drug events among older persons in the ambulatory setting. JAMA 2003; 289(9):1107–16.
23. Budnitz DS, Lovegrove MC, Shehab N, et al. Emergency hospitalizations for adverse drug events in older Americans. N Engl J Med 2011;365(21):2002–12.
24. Budnitz DS, Shehab N, Kegler SR, et al. Medication use leading to emergency department visits for adverse drug events in older adults. Ann Intern Med 2007;147(11):755–65.
25. Thomsen LA, Winterstein AG, Sondergaard B, et al. Systematic review of the incidence and characteristics of preventable adverse drug events in ambulatory care. Ann Pharmacother 2007;41(9):1411–26.
26. Haynes RB, Ackloo E, Sahota N, et al. Interventions for enhancing medication adherence. Cochrane Database Syst Rev 2008;(2):CD000011.
27. Garfinkel D, Mangin D. Feasibility study of a systematic approach for discontinuation of multiple medications in older adults: addressing polypharmacy. Arch Intern Med 2010;170(18):1648–54.
28. Hilmer SN, Gnjidic D, Le Couteur DG. Thinking through the medication list - appropriate prescribing and deprescribing in robust and frail older patients. Aust Fam Physician 2012;41(12):924–8.
29. UptoDate. Available at: http://www.uptodate.com/contents/drug-prescribing-for-older-adults?source=search_result&search=prescribing+Garfinkle&selectedTitle= 1%7E150#H25. Accessed May 30, 2017.
30. Jordan S, Gabe M, Newson L, et al. Medication monitoring for people with dementia in care homes: the feasibility and clinical impact of nurse-led monitoring. ScientificWorldJournal 2014;2014:843621.
31. Cousins D. Current status of the monitoring of medication practice. Am J Health Syst Pharm 2009;66(5 Suppl 3):S49–56.
32. Steinman MA, Miao Y, Boscardin WJ, et al. Prescribing quality in older veterans: a multifocal approach. J Gen Intern Med 2014;29(10):1379–86.
33. Bell SP, Saraf AA. Epidemiology of multimorbidity in older adults with cardiovascular disease. Clin Geriatr Med 2016;32(2):215–26.
34. Downing NS, Shah ND, Neiman JH, et al. Participation of the elderly, women, and minorities in pivotal trials supporting 2011–2013 U.S. Food and Drug Administration approvals. Trials 2016;17(1):199.
35. Boyd CM, Vollenweider D, Puhan MA. Informing evidence-based decision-making for patients with comorbidity: availability of necessary information in clinical trials for chronic diseases. PLoS One 2012;7(8):e41601.

36. Boyd CM, Darer J, Boult C, et al. Clinical practice guidelines and quality of care for older patients with multiple comorbid diseases: implications for pay for performance. JAMA 2005;294(6):716–24.
37. Romera L, Orfila F, Segura JM, et al. Effectiveness of a primary care based multi-factorial intervention to improve frailty parameters in the elderly: a randomised clinical trial: rationale and study design. BMC Geriatr 2014;14:125.
38. Yourman LC, Lee SJ, Schonberg MA, et al. Prognostic indices for older adults: a systematic review. JAMA 2012;307(2):182–92.
39. Min L, Yoon W, Mariano J, et al. The vulnerable elders-13 survey predicts 5-year functional decline and mortality outcomes in older ambulatory care patients. J Am Geriatr Soc 2009;57(11):2070–6.
40. Peron EP, Gray SL, Hanlon JT. Medication use and functional status decline in older adults: a narrative review. Am J Geriatr Pharmacother 2011;9(6):378–91.
41. Hilmer SN, Mager DE, Simonsick EM, et al. Drug burden index score and functional decline in older people. Am J Med 2009;122(12):1142–9.e1-2.
42. Hilmer SN, Gnjidic D. The effects of polypharmacy in older adults. Clin Pharmacol Ther 2009;85(1):86–8.
43. Bennett A, Gnjidic D, Gillett M, et al. Prevalence and impact of fall-risk-increasing drugs, polypharmacy, and drug-drug interactions in robust versus frail hospital-ised falls patients: a prospective cohort study. Drugs Aging 2014;31(3):225–32.
44. Best O, Gnjidic D, Hilmer SN, et al. Investigating polypharmacy and drug burden index in hospitalised older people. Intern Med J 2013;43(8):912–8.
45. Funnell M. What's new in the 2013 guidelines for diabetes care? Nursing 2013; 43(7):66.
46. Nguyen V, deGoma EM, Hossain E, et al. Updated cholesterol guidelines and in-tensity of statin therapy. J Clin Lipidol 2015;9(3):357–9.
47. Armstrong C, Joint National Committe. JNC8 guidelines for the management of hypertension in adults. Am Fam Physician 2014;90(7):503–4.
48. Ickowicz E, American Geriatrics Society Expert Panel on the Care of Older Adults with Multimorbidity. Patient-centered care for older adults with multiple chronic conditions: a stepwise approach from the American Geriatrics Society. J Am Geriatr Soc 2012;60(10):1957–68.
49. Excellencje NBNIfHaC. Medicines Optimisation: the safe and effective use of medicienes to enable the best possible outcomes. NICE guideline NG5. 2015. Available at: https://www.nice.org.uk/guidance/service-delivery–organisation-and-staffing/medicines-management. Accessed February 1, 2017.
50. Paige NM, Nagami GT. The top 10 things nephrologists wish every primary care physician knew. Mayo Clin Proc 2009;84(2):180–6.
51. Antimisiaris D, Miles T, Leey-Casella J, et al. New medical treatments: risks and benefits in practice. Gerontologist 2008;48:303.
52. Hanlon JT, Sloane RJ, Pieper CF, et al. Association of adverse drug reactions with drug-drug and drug-disease interactions in frail older outpatients. Age Ageing 2011;40(2):274–7.
53. Chapple C. Chapter 2: pathophysiology of neurogenic detrusor overactivity and the symptom complex of "Overactive Bladder". Neurourol Urodyn 2014;33: S6–13.
54. Meng E, Lin WY, Lee WC, et al. Pathophysiology of overactive bladder. Low Urin Tract Symptoms 2012;4:48–55.
55. Chancellor MB, Migliaccio-Walle K, Bramley TJ, et al. Long-term patterns of use and treatment failure with anticholinergic agents for overactive bladder. Clin Ther 2013;35(11):1744–51.

56. Schartum-Hansen H, Loland KH, Svingen GF, et al. Use of loop diuretics is associated with increased mortality in patients with suspected coronary artery disease, but without systolic heart failure or renal impairment: an observational study using propensity score matching. PLoS One 2015;10(6):e0124611.
57. Thaler HW, Pienaar S, Wirnsberger G, et al. Bilateral leg edema in an older woman. Z Gerontol Geriatr 2015;48(1):49–51.
58. Ely JW, Osheroff JA, Chambliss ML, et al. Approach to leg edema of unclear etiology. J Am Board Fam Med 2006;19(2):148–60.
59. Casey DA, Antimisiaris D, O'Brien J. Drugs for Alzheimer's disease: are they effective? P T 2010;35(4):208–11.
60. Gopalraj RK, Antimisiaris DE, O'Brien JG, et al. Glossodynia: an unsuspected etiology. J Am Geriatr Soc 2009;57:S119.
61. Paradiso L. Crushing or altering medications: what's happening in residential aged-care facilities? Australas J Ageing 2002;21(3):123–7.
62. Ogawa R, Echizen H. Drug-drug interaction profiles of proton pump inhibitors. Clin Pharmacokinet 2010;49(8):509–33.
63. Miller AD, Smith KM. Medication use in bariatric surgery patients: what orthopedists need to know. Orthopedics 2006;29(2):121–3.
64. Miller AD, Smith KM. Medication and nutrient administration considerations after bariatric surgery. Am J Health Syst Pharm 2006;63(19):1852–7.
65. Shin JM, Sachs G. Pharmacology of proton pump inhibitors. Curr Gastroenterol Rep 2008;10(6):528–34.
66. Sachs G, Shin JM, Howden CW. Review article: the clinical pharmacology of proton pump inhibitors. Aliment Pharmacol Ther 2006;23(Suppl 2):2–8.
67. Louis AJ, Arora VM, Press VG. Evaluating the brief health literacy screen. J Gen Intern Med 2014;29(1):21.
68. Morisky DE, Ang A, Krousel-Wood M, et al. Predictive validity of a medication adherence measure in an outpatient setting. J Clin Hypertens (Greenwich) 2008;10(5):348–54.

Sexuality in the Older Adult

Laura Morton, MD, CMD

KEYWORDS

- Sexuality • Geriatric • Older adult • Sexual dysfunction
- Provider/patient communication

KEY POINTS

- Sexuality is important to older adults, and they continue to be sexually active.
- Sexual response cycles provide a framework for understanding sexuality and dysfunction.
- Anatomic and physiologic changes with aging impact sexual function in both men and women.
- In patients with sexual dysfunction, a thorough medical, psychological, and social evaluation is necessary to diagnose sexual dysfunction and develop a management plan tailored to the underlying cause.
- The topic of sex is not routinely raised in office visits; if providers initiate the conversation, patients are more willing to discuss their sexual concerns.

INTRODUCTION

The population of people older than 65 is increasing more rapidly than all other age groups. There were 46.2 million Americans over the age of 65 in 2014. This number is projected to increase to 82.3 million by 2040 and 90 million by 2060.[1] The health care community will have to adapt and find ways to manage the diverse needs of this increasing part of the population.

Sexuality is an important aspect of a person's life, relationships, and overall quality of life. Sexuality is often addressed in the popular media and social settings. However, health care providers often overlook this topic, especially in the geriatric population. Sexuality has been generally defined as dynamic result of physical ability, drive, attitudes, chances for relationship, and sexual behavior.[2] Sexuality is impacted by physical, psychological, spiritual, and cultural factors. Intimacy describes the characteristic of a relationship comprising feelings of closeness, warmth, and shared life

Disclosure: The author has no commercial or financial conflicts of interest.
Department of Family and Geriatric Medicine, University of Louisville, 501 East Broadway, Suite 240, Louisville, KY 40202, USA
E-mail address: Laura.Morton@louisville.edu

Prim Care Clin Office Pract 44 (2017) 429–438
http://dx.doi.org/10.1016/j.pop.2017.04.004

path. Sexual activity results from the interaction of each partner's physical status, interest, behavior, and attitudes and the underlying quality of the relationship itself and intimacy level.[3,4] Sexuality plays an important role in a person's mental and physical health and quality of life throughout the life spectrum. Therefore, providers should continue to discuss sexuality and sexual concerns with their patients as they age.

MYTHS ABOUT SEXUALITY IN OLDER ADULTS

There are many cultural and societal myths that exist regarding sexuality in older adults. These myths may result from media portrayal of older adults and sexual issues. In a study of medical and psychology students,[5] researchers found that knowledge about aging was strongly linked with knowledge about sexuality. However, knowledge about sexuality and aging was not associated with attitudes, which were more closely related to personal beliefs or social norms.

Many commonly held beliefs about older adults and sexuality have no underlying basis in reality. Common myths regarding older adults and sexuality include sexual activities do not occur (older are asexual), it is humorous, it is filthy ("dirty old man" or "spinster"), older people are too frail for sexual activity, the elderly are not sexually desirable secondary to physical changes.[6–8]

Increasing knowledge about older adults and sexuality and about current sexual practices, will hopefully dispel these myths and improve a provider's ability to address these issues throughout life.

STATISTICS ABOUT SEXUAL ACTIVITY IN OLDER ADULTS

Several studies of older adult sexuality and health in the United States[3,4,9] report that the prevalence of sexual activity with a partner in the last 12 months decreased with increasing age: 73% who were age 57 to 64, 53% who were age 65 to 74, and 26% in those age 75 to 85. In this study, the likelihood of being sexually active was less in women than men across all age groups. Sexually active respondents were more likely to rate their health status positively. In those 75 to 85, 54% of sexually active respondents had intercourse 2 to 3 times per month, and 23% had sex at least once weekly. Seventy percent of men and 50% of women older than age 65 report interest in sex. Other forms of sexual expression were queried, including oral sex and masturbation. In the youngest age group, 58% engaged in oral sex compared with 31% in the oldest group. Masturbation was higher in the younger age group and in men.[9] The frequency of other forms of sexual expression, including hugging, kissing, or sexual touching did not change with age.[3] Availability of a spouse or sexual partner impacts sexuality at older ages. In men 75 to 85, 78% report having a partner; conversely, in women age 75 to 85, 40% report having a partner.[9] This difference may be related to longer life expectancy in women.

Among those sexually active, at least half of the respondents reported at least 1 sexual problem. The most prevalent sexual problems reported in women are lack of interest in sex, trouble with vaginal lubrication, inability to achieve orgasm, finding sex not pleasurable, and pain with sex. For men, the most prevalent sexual problems reported are trouble achieving or maintaining an erection, lack of interest in sex, achieving orgasm too quickly, performance anxiety, and inability to orgasm. In all age groups surveyed, 38% of men and 22% of women reported talking about sex with a physician since age 50.[9]

Given these statistics, it is evident that older adults continue to be interested in sex and that sexuality remains an important part of life.

MODELS OF SEXUAL RESPONSE

The first description of the sexual response cycle was in the landmark work of Masters and Johnson. This model serves as the traditional medical framework for sexual response and to categorize sexual dysfunction. The 4 stages of sexual response are:

1. Excitement: interest or urge for sexual activity
2. Plateau: vascular system and body's response to stimulation
3. Orgasm: climax, height of physiologic response, involuntary
4. Resolution: recovery period after orgasm in which body returns to resting state

The Masters and Johnson model describes sexual response in terms of the body's physiologic response to arousal. Another way of viewing the Masters and Johnson model is that it describes sexuality as a goal-directed experience. In the goal-directed experience, the ultimate goal is intercourse and orgasm. A stepwise foreplay experience (touching, kissing) culminates in intercourse and ultimately orgasm. However, if orgasm is not achieved, there is potential for feelings of failure. Following an algorithm can lead to boredom or limit the sexual experience.[10]

However, a different model captures other important aspects of the sexual experience. In non–goal-directed sexual experience, each act of intimacy is viewed as satisfying on its own; intercourse and orgasm are not essential.[10,11] The cycle of intimacy can be created by partners, and adapted and adjusted throughout each sexual experience, which allows greater flexibility and spontaneity. By viewing sexual experiences in a non–goal-directed manner, there is no specific path to follow, and any part of the process can be repeated or skipped, depending on the moment and desires of the participants. The non–goal-directed sexual model incorporates the psychological and emotional aspects of sexual experiences and the intimacy shared by the partners.

FEMALE SEXUAL PHYSIOLOGY AND CHANGES WITH AGING

Physiologic sexual response that occurs in women does exhibit changes with aging. If pathologic or comorbid conditions are present, these can greatly impact female sexual response. During the excitement phase, there is decreased vaginal blood flow, genital engorgement, and lubrication. The plateau phase is prolonged and there is less color change of the labia. Women maintain their capacity for multiple orgasms. However, weaker and less frequent contractions of the perineal muscles occur. During the resolution phase, there is a more rapid loss of vasocongestion than in younger years.[12]

Female Sexual Physiology and Changes with Aging: Endocrine System

Loss of estrogen with menopause is a significant physiologic event that can affect various aspects of women's sexual function. The median age of menopause in the United States is 51 years. Given that the average life expectancy of women is 81.2 years,[13] women will spend approximately 30 years after menopause. Low levels of estrogen lead to changes within the genitourinary tract, including[12]

- Shortening of the vagina
- Vaginal dryness
- Changes in the bacterial flora and pH balance
- Thinning of the labia
- Decrease in fat pad under mons pubis

This urogenital atrophy makes the vaginal mucosa more susceptible to trauma from sexual activity, potentially leading to dyspareunia and vaginal bleeding. There is also increased risk of urinary tract infections and urinary incontinence secondary to changes in urethral epithelium. Urogenital atrophy is treated with localized topical application of estrogen.[6,13]

With decreased ovarian function, there is a decrease in production of androgens and dehydroepiandrosterone, which can impact libido, arousal, genital sensation, and orgasm. There is currently no US Food and Drug Administration–approved treatment for androgen insufficiency in women.[12]

Female Sexual Physiology and Changes with Aging: Vascular System

The urogenital vascular system plays an important role in female sexual response. The genital microvasculature is instrumental in genital sensation and orgasm. Vaginal lubrication is produced by congestion of blood vessels within the vaginal walls during sexual stimulation. With atherosclerosis, there is a delay in vaginal engorgement and loss of lubrication. Atherosclerotic disease also leads to decreased vaginal and clitoral sensation and orgasm.[12]

Female Sexual Physiology and Changes with Aging: Musculoskeletal System

With aging, changes in the musculoskeletal system related to flexibility and mobility of the lower extremities can lead to difficulty with some sexual positions. To address these issues, alternative sexual positions can be explored, including partners lying on their sides or using furniture to assist with positioning. Pelvic musculature changes can lead to weaker contraction and relaxation of perineal muscles during sexual arousal and orgasm.[12]

Female Sexual Physiology and Changes with Aging: Genitourinary System

Genitourinary system changes happen because of the decrease in estrogen. This can lead to urogenital atrophy and prolapse of the uterus and vaginal tissues. These anatomic changes can interfere with penetration and cause pain with intercourse. Pessaries can be used to treat prolapse but are not always successful and are difficult for some women to use. Surgical procedures to correct prolapse may improve sexual function for some women.

Urinary incontinence can occur and often leads to psychological or physical discomfort with sexual intercourse. Treatment of urinary incontinence involves treating the underlying condition and may improve sexual functioning.[12]

FEMALE SEXUAL DYSFUNCTION

Several classification systems exist for female sexual dysfunction, including the Diagnostic and Statistical Manual of Mental Disorders, Fifth Edition; International Classification of Diseases, 10th Edition; and Consensus Statement from the Fourth International Consultation on Sexual Medicine.[12,14] Sexual dysfunction can be categorized as follows: sexual desire disorder, sexual arousal disorder, orgasmic disorder, vaginismus, and dyspareunia.[12]

In older adult women, the cause of sexual dysfunction can be primary or secondary and includes psychological, physical, or social factors.[12] Examples of secondary causes of sexual dysfunction include depression (psychological), physical debility or urinary incontinence and related anxiety (physical), and social factors, such as guilt related to relationships after the loss of a spouse. To determine the etiology of the sexual dysfunction, it is important to obtain a thorough history and perform a focused physical examination. The history should include the timing, severity, frequency, and duration of the sexual concern. To better understand the setting in which the sexual problems occur, it is important to also understand the social setting, the characteristics of the relationship, medications, over-the-counter medications, and substance use. Medications commonly associated with female sexual dysfunction include selective serotonin inhibitors, antipsychotics, mood stabilizers (eg, lithium), phenytoin, digoxin, clonidine, and opioids.[12,15] During this process, the information about the partner's health, physical, and mental functioning should be obtained.

Treatment of sexual dysfunction should be based on treating the underlying causes of the sexual dysfunction. An interdisciplinary approach is useful to address these complex issues in a holistic, person-centered manner, including psychosocial and medical issues. Couples therapy and sex therapy can address interpersonal and relationship issues. Pelvic physical therapy helps women with pelvic floor dysfunction and aid in those with dyspareunia. Lifestyle changes, including diet and exercise, promote improvement of body image. Topical estrogens and lubricants are used for the treatment of urogenital atrophy. Systemic hormone replacement therapy (HRT) remains controversial in the treatment of female sexual dysfunction because of the lack of certainty regarding its role in prevention or promotion of adverse cardiovascular effects.[16] There are no US Food and Drug Administration–approved medications for the treatment of female sexual dysfunction.[12] Given the population changes and importance of sexual function to quality of life, hopefully more treatments will be developed to manage female sexual dysfunction.

MALE SEXUAL PHYSIOLOGY AND CHANGES WITH AGING

In the Massachusetts Male Aging Study,[17] men were surveyed and followed up over 9 years regarding their sexual activity. At the end of the 9-year period, the average frequency of intercourse declined by almost 2 times per month, and the average number of erections decreased by 8 times per month. The frequency of ejaculation with masturbation did not change during the study.

There are changes in male sexual physiology that occur with aging. There is a gradual slowing of physical reaction time to stimulation; more time is required for arousal, to complete the sexual activity, and to become aroused again for sexual activity.[18,19] Erections may become somewhat less firm with age, which may be caused by the decrease in elastic fibers, collagen, and smooth muscle in the penis.[8] Despite these changes in erections, they usually retain the capacity for intercourse. There is also lower production of semen and ejaculatory volume. Ejaculation is less forceful with aging. Orgasm may be shorter in duration, less intense, and characterized by decreased urethral and prostatic contractions. After orgasm, there is rapid detumescence and testicular descent. The refractory period is prolonged. Male fertility usually diminishes in the mid-70s, but may continue into the 90s.[8,18,19]

MALE SEXUAL DYSFUNCTION

There are 4 primary types of male sexual dysfunction in older adults: erectile dysfunction (ED), decreased desire, psychological issues (including performance anxiety), and inability to achieve orgasm.[14,15,18,19] Decreased desire or libido can occur for multiple reasons, including general health, decreased levels of testosterone, or psychosocial concerns. Performance anxiety occurs when men become preoccupied with performance and masculinity to such an extent that those thoughts lead to sexual difficulties. This can be seen in widower's syndrome, in which an older man in a new relationship feels guilt and develops sexual dysfunction secondary to his perceived unfaithfulness to his deceased spouse. Inability to orgasm or to achieve ejaculation can occur.[18,19]

Erectile Dysfunction: Prevalence and Definition

ED, the inability to obtain or maintain an erection adequate for intercourse, is the most prevalent type of sexual dysfunction in older men, ranging from 31% to 44%.[3,9,17] In the Massachusetts Male Aging Study, the probably of ED at age 40 was 40% and 70% at age 70.[17] Erectile dysfunction, although common, is not a part of normal aging. A diagnosis of ED should not be made until it occurs in greater than 25% of the encounters with the same sexual partner.

Erectile Dysfunction: Vascular Etiology

The most common etiology of ED is vascular disease, which results in arterial insufficiency or venous leakage. With atherosclerotic disease, there is decreased blood flow to the lacunar spaces within the corpora cavernosum, which is necessary for vasodilation and filling to achieve erection. Atherosclerosis may also cause ischemia, leading to replacement of smooth muscle by connective tissue.[18–20]

Venous disease, either occlusion or leakage, leads to difficulty with erection, as erection requires blood to be stored in the corpus cavernosum through compression of emissary veins. This condition can result from Peyronie disease, arteriovenous fistula, or trauma. With aging, there is an increase in the size and number of the venous outflow paths. There is also decreased compliance and inability to expand the trabeculae against the tunica albuginea.[18–20]

Erectile Dysfunction: Neurologic Etiology

Neurologic disease is the second most common cause of ED and can cause peripheral or central neurologic erectile issues. This condition can result from diseases that affect parasympathetic spinal cord or peripheral efferent autonomic fibers to the penis, leading to impaired penile smooth muscle relaxation and prevention of vasodilation necessary for erection. Diabetes mellitus and neuropathy can cause peripheral autonomic dysfunction. Local nerve damage from surgery or trauma can also lead to ED. Stroke, Parkinson disease, and depression are central neurologic causes of ED.[18,20]

Erectile Dysfunction: Endocrine Etiology

Hormonal changes in aging men include decreased function of the hypothalamic-pituitary-gonadal axis and decreased testosterone. With androgen deficiency, there can be reduced libido, decreased sensation in the penis, erectile dysfunction, and decreased orgasm.[18,20] As with women's systemic HRT, male HRT is also controversial because of concerns about the use of testosterone replacement in older adults with known cardiovascular disease. Significant andropause occurs in 20% of men in their 60s and 50% of men in their 80s, and testosterone levels decrease in men by 1% every year after age 30.[21] Consequently, HRT is common in a variety of ages and poses higher risk to those with multiple chronic diseases, especially cardiovascular disease. "A detailed discussion of clinical practice guidelines about hormone replacement therapy (see Bradley R. Williams and Janet Soojeung Cho's articles, "Hormone Replacement: The Fountain of Youth?" in this issue)."

Erectile Dysfunction: Systemic Diseases

Many medical illnesses are associated with erectile dysfunction. With diabetes mellitus, the prevalence of ED is 75%. More than 50% of men have ED within 10 years of the diagnosis of diabetes.[18–20] Diabetes can decrease blood flow and cause neurologic damage, which leads to difficulty with erections.

Vascular and neurologic diseases are commonly associated with erectile dysfunction. Chronic obstructive pulmonary disease and obstructive sleep apnea are associated with ED through low testosterone levels secondary to chronic hypoxia and respond to treatment with testosterone.[22]

Alcoholism can lead to ED by leading to increased levels of estrogen and decreased levels of testosterone.[15,20] In patients with liver disease, there is testicular atrophy, gynecomastia, and increased sexual dysfunction. Testosterone supplementation in alcoholism is usually not effective treatment of erectile dysfunction.[22] Smoking and substance abuse also lead to ED through impairment of blood flow. Physical activity can decrease the likelihood of or improve erectile dysfunction.[18]

Male Sexual Dysfunction: Evaluation

Once sexual dysfunction has been diagnosed, it is essential to obtain a thorough history and physical to determine the likely etiology and develop an appropriate management plan. The history should include information about the following[18–20]:

- Sexual history: duration of sexual issues, quality of erections (nocturnal, with masturbation, or with intercourse), differences with partners
- Psychosocial history: partner or partners, significant life changes, depression, anxiety
- Medical history: comorbid medical conditions (stable, unstable)
- Iatrogenic: any surgery, trauma, other potentially reversible causes
- Medications: prescription, over-the-counter medications, or medications that may interfere with ED treatment

The physical examination is also important and should assess the genitourinary system, endocrine systems, blood pressure, femoral and pedal pulses, and a thorough neurologic examination. In most cases, the etiology of sexual dysfunction can be determined through the history and physical examination.

There are often historical clues that suggest certain diagnoses. Rapid onset of ED usually indicates psychogenic causes or genitourinary trauma or surgery. A history of nonsustained erection is suggestive of anxiety or vascular steal. With pelvic steal, blood flow is redirected from the penis to buttocks during thrusting. This can be managed with position changes, side-to-side sexual position or the unaffected partner on top. If there is a history of depression or substance use, then the sexual dysfunction is likely related to these issues. With underlying psychogenic causes, nocturnal erections still occur. If there is complete loss of nocturnal erections, this suggests underlying vascular disease or neurologic disease.[20]

Male Sexual Dysfunction: Treatment

Treatments of male sexual dysfunction should be started in a stepwise manner from least invasive to more invasive therapy. First, psychosocial treatment, vacuum erection devices, and constriction band devices can be used. If these are not effective, then pharmacologic treatment can be initiated. Phosphodiesterase type 5 inhibitors are approved by the US Food and Drug Administration for the treatment of erectile dysfunction. These medications are not erectogenic and require sexual stimulation to work. Phosphodiesterase type 5 inhibitors are contraindicated with nitrates because they potentiate hypotensive effects of nitrates. Adverse effects include headache, flushing, and visual disturbance.[20] Patients should be advised to allow more than one attempt of the medication before declaring treatment failure.

If the less-invasive options are not effective, intracavernous or transurethral vasoactive agents can be effective. These erectogenic agents are effective but require injection or insertion of a urethral suppository. Hypotension is a possible adverse effect.[20] Penile prostheses can be implanted for severe refractory erectile dysfunction but are expensive and the most invasive treatment option.[20]

Selection of effective treatments for patients with male sexual dysfunction requires an understanding of the underlying etiology, the patient's preferences and goals for sexual function, and an awareness of the patient's functional ability. With this information, providers can select and then escalate therapy from nonpharmacologic to pharmacologic and lastly more invasive modalities to manage male sexual dysfunction. Frail, medically complex patients are best treated with nonpharmacologic methods given potential interactions and adverse medication effects. Invasive therapies for ED should only be considered after other treatment methods have proven unsuccessful and then only in patients who are physically capable of undergoing those procedures.

PROVIDER/PATIENT INTERACTIONS

Sexuality in the older adult is a multifaceted subject that requires a holistic, person-centered approach. However, the topic of older adult sexuality remains a challenge in current medical practice. In a study by Lindau and colleagues,[9] 38% of men and 22% of women reported having discussed sex with a physician since the age of 50. A study by Nusbaum and colleagues[23] addressed the sexual health care needs of women older than 65, especially patient/provider communication. For 68% of the women in the study, sexuality had never arisen during an office visit. Older women were less likely than younger women to have had the topic of sex raised during an office visit (33% vs 52%). When sex was raised during the visit, older women were twice as likely as the physician to have raised the topic. Of those surveyed, 97% said they would have discussed their sexual concerns had the physician asked. The older and younger women reported that it was easier to discuss concerns about sexuality if the physician raised the topic. Patient-related barriers to discussion of sexual issues include embarrassment (patients prefer talking with a provider of similar age and sex) and adequate time for the discussion. Providers appearing rushed hindered the discussion of sexual issues. Eighty percent of the women surveyed were willing to return for another appointment specifically dedicated to their sexual concerns.[23]

Providers are also reluctant to initiate discussions about sexuality. Provider barriers include[23]:

- Believing the stereotype that older adults are asexual
- Fear of offending patients
- Lack of confidence in own skills to discuss sexual issues
- Not having adequate time for the discussion
- Provider discomfort with the subject matter
- Provider seeming uninterested or impersonal

Given the importance of the topic of sexuality in older adults, providers and patients must work together to improve discussions about sexual concerns. To improve discussions of sexuality with patients, providers should:

- Exhibit professional demeanor
- Be comfortable with subject of sex
- Be understanding and empathetic
- Inquire about the sexual function of the patient's partner
- Raise sexual health topic routinely, as in routine wellness
- Use sexuality/sexual function questionnaire form in routine patient history forms

- Use open-ended questions
  - Many of my patients with similar conditions have questions about sexual function and how their disease impacts sexuality. What concerns do you have?
  - Are you sexually active? Then ask for clarification of answers.
  - Is a physical relationship an important part of your life? Are there any areas that you are interested in improving?
  - For patients in nursing home or group living situation: Finding time alone may be difficult in your current living situation. Is this a problem for you and your partner?

Improving discussions with patients about sexuality will facilitate provider-patient rapport and enhance the sexual care of older adults.

SUMMARY

Sexuality is an important part of a person's life, continuing into older age. Sexuality is not traditionally discussed in the health care setting, even though patients express an interest in discussing the topic if the provider initiates the conversation. With aging, there are physiologic changes that occur that can impact sexual function. Other comorbid conditions can exacerbate other underlying sexual issues. To diagnose sexual dysfunction, providers must obtain a thorough history and physical examination, including psychosocial factors. The underlying etiology of the sexual dysfunction serves as the basis for a person-centered management plan to address the patient's concerns. To improve the overall care of older adults with sexual concerns, providers should initiate discussions with their patients, listen, and work with patients to create a plan.

REFERENCES

1. A Profile of Older Americans: 2015. Administration on Aging. Administration for Community Living. U.S. Department of Health and Human Services. 2016. Available at: http://www.aoa.acl.gov/aging_statistics/profile/2015/docs/2015-Profile.pdf. Accessed October 27, 2016.
2. Lindau ST, Laumann EO, Levinson W, et al. Synthesis of scientific disciplines in pursuit of health: The Interactive Biopsychosocial Model. Perspect Biol Med 2003;46:S74–86.
3. Waite LJ, Laumann EO, Das A, et al. Sexuality: measures of partnerships, practices, attitudes, and problems in the national social life, health, and aging study. J Gerontol B Psychol Sci Soc Sci 2009;64B(S1):i56–66.
4. Galinsky AM, McClintock MK, Waite LJ. Sexuality and physical contact in national social life, health, and aging project wave 2. J Gerontol B Psychol Sci Soc Sci 2014;69(8):S83–98.
5. Snyder RJ, Zweig RA. Medical and psychology students' knowledge and attitudes regarding aging and sexuality. Gerontol Geriatr Educ 2010;31:235–55.
6. Ginsberg TB. Aging and sexuality. Med Clin North Am 2006;90:1025–36.
7. Kessel B. Sexuality in the older person. Age Ageing 2001;30:121–4.
8. Lochlainn MN, Kenny RA. Sexual activity and aging. J Am Med Dir Assoc 2013; 14:565–72.
9. Lindau ST, Schumm LP, Laumann EO, et al. A study of sexuality and health among older adults in the United States. N Engl J Med 2007;357:762–74.
10. Timmers RL, Sinclair LG, James JR. Treating goal-directed intimacy. Soc Work 1976;21(5):491–2.

11. Basson R. The female sexual response: a different model. J Sex Marital Ther 2000;26(1):51–65.
12. Lindau S. Chapter 47. Sexuality, sexual function, and the aging woman. In: Halter JB, Ouslander JG, Tinetti ME, et al, editors. Hazzard's geriatric medicine and gerontology. 6th edition. New York: McGraw-Hill; 2009. Available at: http://accessmedicine.mhmedical.com.echo.louisville.edu/content.aspx?bookid=371&Sectionid=41587658. Accessed October 29, 2016.
13. Kochanek MA, Murphy SL, Xu J, et al. Deaths: final data for 2014. Natl Vital Stat Rep 2016;65(4):1–122. Available at: http://www.cdc.gov/nchs/data/nvsr/nvsr65/nvsr65_04.pdf. Accessed October 28, 2016.
14. McCabe MP, Sharlip ID, Atalla E, et al. Definitions of sexual dysfunctions in women and men: a consensus statement from the Fourth International Consultation on Sexual Medicine 2015. Sex Med 2016;13:135–43.
15. Hillman JL. Clinical perspectives on elderly sexuality. New York: Kluwer Academic; 2000.
16. Yang X, Reckelhoff J. Estrogen, hormonal replacement therapy and cardiovascular disease. Curr Opin Nephrol Hypertens 2011;20(2):133–8.
17. Araujo AB, Mohr BA, McKinlay JB. Changes in sexual function in middle-aged and older men: longitudinal data from the Massachusetts Male Aging Study. J Am Geriatr Soc 2004;52:1502–9.
18. Tenover J. Chapter 49. Sexuality, sexual function, androgen therapy, and the aging male. In: Halter JB, Ouslander JG, Tinetti ME, et al, editors. Hazzard's geriatric medicine and gerontology. 6th edition. New York: McGraw-Hill; 2009. Available at: http://accessmedicine.mhmedical.com.echo.louisville.edu/content.aspx?bookid=371&Sectionid=41587660. Accessed October 28, 2016.
19. Gentili A, Godschalk M. Sexual health & dysfunction. In: Williams BA, Chang A, Ahalt C, et al, editors. Current diagnosis & treatment: geriatrics. 2nd edition. New York: McGraw-Hill; 2014. Available at: http://accessmedicine.mhmedical.com.echo.louisville.edu/content.aspx?bookid=953&Sectionid=53375670. Accessed October 26, 2016.
20. Seftel AD. From aspiration to achievement: assessment and noninvasive treatment of erectile dysfunction in aging men. J Am Geriatr Soc 2005;53:119–30.
21. Brawer M. Testosterone replacement in men with andropause: an overview. Rev Urol 2004;6(suppl 6):S9–15.
22. Morley JE, Tariq SH. Sexuality and disease. Clin Geriatr Med 2003;19:563–73.
23. Nusbaum MR, Singh AR, Pyles AA. Sexual healthcare needs of women aged 65 and older. J Am Geriatr Soc 2004;52(1):117–22.

Dementia for the Primary Care Provider

Daniela Claudia Moga, MD, PhD[a,b,*], Monica Roberts, PharmD[c],
Gregory Jicha, MD, PhD[d]

KEYWORDS

- Dementia • Mild cognitive impairment • Psychiatric symptoms • Risk factors
- Treatment

KEY POINTS

- Dementia, a significant and growing public health problem, poses an important burden on patients, caregivers, and society as a whole.
- Primary care providers (PCPs) should treat dementia as a chronic health condition playing a key role in diagnosis and providing comprehensive care for patients with this diagnosis.
- Routine diagnosis should include work-up for reversible medical and nondegenerative causes for dementia that are common in the elderly, in addition to identifying degenerative causes for decline.
- Treatment should be multimodal, including management of cognitive decline as well as comorbid behavioral and psychiatric symptoms of dementia, using nonpharmacologic approaches to care as first-line treatment.

INTRODUCTION

Dementia and prodromal memory loss (mild cognitive impairment [MCI]), defined as major and mild neurocognitive disorders (NCDs), respectively, based on *Diagnostic and Statistical Manual of Mental Disorders* (Fifth Edition) (*DSM-5*) terminology, represent one of the most important and growing public health issues facing society today.[1,2] Abnormal cognitive decline in the aging population suggestive of dementia in its active or prodromal forms is distinct from normal age-related changes in cognition and should be recognized as such.

Disclosures: No relevant relationships to disclose.
[a] Department of Pharmacy Practice and Science, College of Pharmacy, University of Kentucky, 789 South Limestone Street, Room 241, Lexington, KY 40536-0596, USA; [b] Department of Epidemiology, College of Public Health, University of Kentucky, 789 South Limestone Street, Room 241, Lexington, KY 40536-0596, USA; [c] College of Pharmacy, University of Kentucky, 789 South Limestone Street, Room 241, Lexington, KY 40536, USA; [d] Department of Neurology, University of Kentucky, UK Medical Center MN 150- Lexington, KY 40536, USA
* Corresponding author. Department of Pharmacy Practice and Science, College of Pharmacy, University of Kentucky, 789 South Limestone, Room 241, Lexington, KY 40536.
E-mail address: daniela.moga@uky.edu

Prim Care Clin Office Pract 44 (2017) 439–456
http://dx.doi.org/10.1016/j.pop.2017.04.005

A key feature of dementia is impairment or loss of cognitive functions leading to impairments in normal activities and relationships. Individuals diagnosed with dementia are generally impaired in at least 2 areas of cognitive function, including but not limited to memory, communication and language, ability to focus and pay attention, reasoning and judgment, and visual perception.[3] In addition to memory loss, patients with dementia often lose their ability to maintain emotional control, leading to personality changes, behavioral problems, and overt psychiatric features, including depression, anxiety, agitation, delusions, hallucinations, sleep disturbances, and motor restlessness.[4] Advances in understanding of dementia have allowed even earlier recognition of individuals at risk for functional decline as a result of abnormal cognitive impairment.

Individuals with abnormal cognitive impairment who are able to compensate for their cognitive symptoms can often retain normal functional activities for a period of time and meet criteria for MCI (minor NCD).[1] Thus, the transition from normal aging to MCI is dependent on cognitive decline, whereas the distinction between MCI and dementia is dependent on the cognitive impairment progressing to the point where normal activities of daily living (ADLs) are impaired (**Fig. 1**).[5] Identification of persons with MCI allows early evaluation for medical causes of decline that may be reversible or indicate an alternative treatment strategy, and, importantly, for the identification of those at risk for further decline and eventual functional impairment.[6,7]

EPIDEMIOLOGY
Incidence and Prevalence Estimates

Dementia affects more than 5.5 million Americans of all ages and an estimated 13% of Americans age 65 years and older (**Fig. 2**A).[2] A recent epidemiologic study from Olmsted County, Minnesota, estimated the prevalence of MCI in the population 65 years or older at 16%.[8,9] Despite the prevalence of MCI and dementia in the aging population, fewer than half of such patients are diagnosed in the primary care setting if at all.[2] These data illustrate a key point, that almost 1 of every 3 patients seen in primary care has some degree of cognitive impairment that may not be recognized, investigated, or treated in many cases (**Fig. 2**B).

Risk Factors

The strongest risk factor for dementia is advanced age. The overall prevalence of dementia is 1% to 2% at age 65 years and increases to 30% at age 85 years.[2,3] Although the prevalence of dementia is higher in women than in men, this is likely attributable to the longer average lifespan of women rather than to any true biologic effect of gender.[2] Some forms of dementia, such as Parkinson disease dementia and dementia with Lewy bodies, have a true gender disposition, affecting men 3 times more often than women.[10]

Family history is known to increase risk of dementia, and genetic markers related to specific types of dementia have been identified.[2] Although true autosomal inheritance

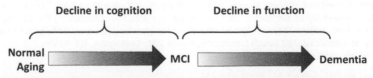

Fig. 1. Schematic of transitions from normal aging to MCI and further to dementia dependent on both cognitive decline as well as loss of function.

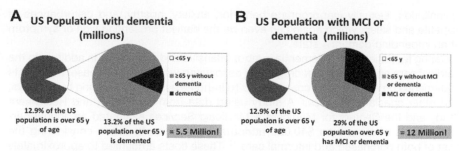

Fig. 2. Population estimates of (*A*) dementia and (*B*) MCI or dementia in the United States demonstrate that almost 1 of 3 seniors have some degree of abnormal cognitive impairment that should be addressed medically. (*Data from* Alzheimer's Association. 2017 Alzheimer's disease facts and figures. Alzheimers Dement 2017;13(4):325–74; and Petersen RC, Roberts RO, Knopman DS, et al. Prevalence of mild cognitive impairment is higher in men. The Mayo Clinic study of aging. Neurology 2010;75(10):889–97.)

is found in all forms of dementia, most genetic and familial predisposition is related to genes that modify risk rather than confer absolute determination of future disease state. Although many genetic tests are available clinically, the American Academy of Neurology practice parameter recommends that genetic testing be avoided, unless there is a suspicion of autosomal dominant disease to limit the potential social, psychological, financial, and legal repercussions of being identified as a carrier of a risk gene for the future development of dementia.[3]

Alongside continuing breakthroughs in understanding of the genetic disposition for the development of discrete dementia states, environmental risk factors, such as medical comorbidities, traumatic and or toxic exposures, and many other lifestyle factors are also recognized to play an important role in conferring risk for dementia.[4,11] Most experts concede that dementia is likely the result of multifactorial processes, including environmental risks, such as head trauma, smoking, sedentary lifestyle, poor diet, low mental activity, social isolation, and suboptimal control of multiple chronic health conditions, such as diabetes, hypertension, and hyperlipidemia.[4,11]

Despite recognition of these modifiable environmental risks, a recent consensus panel convened by the National Institutes of Health concluded that there is limited evidence that any intervention targeting these risk factors may be helpful in delaying the onset of or avoiding dementia for those destined to develop a degenerative disease.[11] Although many investigators have attributed this lack of evidence to poorly designed trials that may be targeting the wrong life stage for intervention (ie, midlife, not late-life hypertension, is a risk for dementia), there exists a wealth of scientifically and medically plausible data supporting risk factor modification as a strategy for lessening dementia burden in the population today.[4] Ongoing work in this area is needed to resolve this debate.[11]

Disease Burden

Patients with dementia experience both cognitive and neuropsychiatric symptoms that evolve and progress over time. Memory loss is often an early cognitive symptom in Alzheimer disease, although impairments in executive function, language, judgment, and spatial abilities develop unpredictably or may even be the presenting sign or symptom in many cases of dementia resulting from other degenerative disease states.[1,2,4] Complicating the cognitive effects of dementia are neuropsychiatric symptoms, such as depression, suicidal ideation, hallucinations, delusions, agitation, disinhibition, sexually inappropriate behavior, anxiety, apathy, and disturbances of appetite and sleep, which again can even be the earliest presenting sign or symptom of an impending dementia state.[1,2,4]

Caring for patients with dementia is labor intensive and expensive. In addition to the medical care and prescription drug costs associated with chronic disease, the effects of dementia on ADLs lead to costs related to in-home assistance, nursing home stays, and other specialty services.[2] A study using data from the Health and Retirement Study and the Centers for Medicare & Medicaid Services estimated an annual per-patient cost of more than $40,000 attributable to dementia when considering the cost of both purchased and informal care.[12] These costs amounted to approximately $259 billion nationwide in 2016 and are expected to more than quadruple to $1.1 trillion by 2050 due to the aging of the US population.[2]

For health care professionals, dementia and the comorbidities common to elderly populations present a complex challenge that benefits from interprofessional collaborative care teams. Comprehensive management of dementia may require the expertise of geriatricians, psychiatrists, social workers, pharmacists, and other professionals.[2] PCPs may need to use innovative care models to ensure coordination among providers and caregivers and improve outcomes for dementia patients.[2] The costs of care for those with dementia often can be augmented by compromised management of other chronic health care conditions as a result of cognitive interference with scheduled management of such conditions. Thus, it is imperative for PCPs to recognize dementia to ensure adequate, stable care not only of the dementia but also for optimal management of patients' other chronic health conditions, such as diabetes and hypertension, among others.

DEMENTIA DIAGNOSIS AND PRIMARY CARE SETTINGS
Standard Diagnosis

All forms of dementia share the common clinical feature of an acquired (ie, not developmental) deficit in cognitive, behavioral, or psychiatric function.[1-4] These exclude mental disorders that may have comorbid cognitive deficits but not as a core clinical feature (eg, schizophrenia, bipolar disorder, and major depressive disorder).[1,3,4] Therefore, a major NDC (dementia) diagnosis should be considered only after conducting differential diagnosis with delirium, or mental disorders like schizophrenia or major depressive disorder. The major NCD diagnosis is based on the cognitive decline (on one or more cognitive domains) that interferes with the ability for living an independent life and perform everyday activities. This cognitive decline can be described by the individual, a close informant, or a clinician. Standardized neuropsychological tests are needed to document the impairment in cognitive performance and to evaluate cognitive status following diagnosis.[1] Diagnostic criteria for mild NCD (MCI) are similar, with the exceptions that cognitive decline is modest and the deficits do not interfere with a patient's capacity for independence.[1,5]

Diagnosis of dementia should include consideration of etiologic cause, including Alzheimer disease, frontotemporal lobar degeneration, Lewy body disease, vascular disease, traumatic brain injury, substance/medication use, HIV infection, prion disease, Parkinson disease, Huntington disease, another medical condition, multiple etiologies, or unspecified.[1-5] More detailed diagnostic criteria for each subtype are available in **Table 1**.[1] Additional specifiers for NCD include with/without behavioral disturbance and severity of impact on ADLs.[1]

Given these diagnostic criteria, there are 4 primary considerations that should be included as part of every patient's evaluation and workup, including (1) establishing

Table 1 Types of dementia		
Dementia Type	**Brain Pathology**	**Key Features**
Alzheimer disease	β-Amyloid plaques outside neurons and tau protein inside neurons eventually lead to neuron dysfunction and death	• Most common type, accounting for up to 60%–80% of dementia cases alone or as part of mixed dementia • Early signs include memory loss disrupting daily life, difficulties in planning or completing routine tasks, confusion, impacted judgment, and change in personality and mood. • In later stages, may cause behavior changes, disorientation, and difficulty speaking, swallowing, and walking • Please refer to the "10 Early Signs and Symptoms of Alzheimer's" material developed by the Alzheimer's Association (http://alz.org/10-signs-symptoms-alzheimers-dementia.asp)
Vascular dementia	Blockage or damage to vessels in the brain cause strokes that affect functioning	• Often coexists with Alzheimer disease • Early signs likely to include impaired judgment, planning, and decision making; may have motor function deficiencies, such as slow gait and poor balance or language impairment, depending on location of vascular injury • Focal neurologic signs and symptoms as well as brain imaging demonstrating significant cerebrovascular injury are key indicators. • Location and extent of brain injuries determine specific manifestation of dementia and/or other impairment.
Dementia with Lewy bodies	Alpha-synuclein aggregations in neurons of the cerebral cortex	• Early signs likely to include dream enactment behavior, visual hallucinations, visuospatial impairment, parkinsonian features, and marked cognitive fluctuations, possibly in the absence of memory deficits • Cognitive and psychiatric symptoms occur at least 1 year prior to onset of significant parkinsonism and motor deficits
Frontotemporal lobar degeneration/ frontotemporal dementia	Frontal and temporal lobes atrophy; upper layers of cortex soften and show protein accumulation	• Accounts for 10% of dementia cases; symptoms typically develop at earlier age (45–60 y). • Early signs include personality and behavioral changes (behavioral variant) • Or difficulty producing or understanding language (language variants, including primary progressive aphasia or semantic dementia
Parkinson disease dementia	Alpha-synuclein aggregations in substantia nigra	• Movement disorder with early symptoms including rigidity, tremor, and gait changes • Progresses to dementia with signs and symptoms similar to those seen in dementia with Lewy bodies • Parkinsonism occurs at least 1 year prior to cognitive decline.

(continued on next page)

Table 1
(continued)

Dementia Type	Brain Pathology	Key Features
Prion disease	Prions cause misfolding and malfunction of other proteins throughout brain	• Rapidly fatal with memory and coordination deficits and behavioral changes • Very rare; may occur due to genetics, infection, or unknown cause • Creutzfeldt-Jakob disease thought to be caused by infected beef products (mad cow disease)
Normal pressure hydrocephalus	Build-up of fluid in the brain caused by impaired reabsorption of CSF	• Accounts for <5% of dementia cases; increased risk if history of brain hemorrhage or meningitis • Difficulty walking, attentional impairment, and inability to control urination • May require installation of shunt in the brain to drain fluid
Mixed dementias	Pathologic evidence of more than 1 cause of dementia	• Approximately half of older people with dementia show abnormalities associated with multiple causes. • Risk of multiple dementia types increases with age

Adapted from Alzheimer's Association. 2017 Alzheimer's disease facts and figures. Alzheimers Dement 2017;13(4):325–74; with permission.

a level of cognitive performance and convincing evidence (history or longitudinal examination) that this represents a change from past level of performance; (2) exploring any potential functional decline that may help classify the cognitive impairment as mild NCD (MCI), without loss of function, or major NCD (dementia), with significant loss of function; (3) investigating medical comorbidities and confounders that may be responsible for the cognitive and or functional decline seen—this includes a standard work-up for potentially reversible medical causes of dementia; and (4) investigating other potential psychiatric comorbidities or causative processes.[3,4] There are a variety of tools that have been well validated to assist in each of these steps, but the ultimate diagnosis remains clinical, based often on pure sound clinical judgment rather than any single abnormal test result.[1–4]

Neuropsychological testing serves as a primary tool in the diagnosis of dementia and MCI.[1–5] This could include simple cognitive screening measures, more comprehensive bedside testing, or in some cases full neuropsychological evaluation. A patient's performance on any particular test should be compared with norms appropriate to age, education, and cultural background. Major NCD (dementia) is typically diagnosed when a patient tests at the 3rd percentile or below, and mild NCD (MCI) between the 3rd and 16th percentiles (**Fig. 3**A).[1] Such statistical definitions taken out of context in regard to decline from previous levels of performance result in misdiagnosing one-sixth of the population who may be chronically below the 16th percentile. It may be more sensitive to establish change from baseline for higher performing individuals looking for change in cognitive testing at the 1.5 SD level for earlier detection of transition to MCI or dementia (**Fig. 3**B).[4,5] In addition to aiding in diagnosis, testing can establish baseline cognitive function and determine disease severity both at diagnosis and as dementia progresses.[4] The diagnosis of cognitive decline should be based on both subjective and objective evidence. *DSM-5* notes that an exclusive focus on cognitive testing may delay diagnosis in a high-functioning

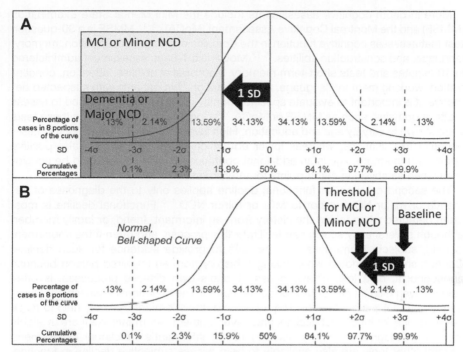

Fig. 3. (A) MCI or minor NCD is characterized by performance in the lowest 16th percentile (<1 SD below the mean), whereas dementia or major NCD is characterized by performance in the lowest 3rd percentile (<1.5 SD below the mean). (B) Change greater than 1 SD from baseline is sufficient to diagnose cognitive impairment in the MCI or minor NCD range even if the absolute score remains in the normal range. (*Data from* American Psychiatric Association. Diagnostic and statistical manual of mental disorders: DSM-V. Washington, DC: APA Press; 2013; with permission.)

individual or misdiagnose a patient whose impaired performance does not represent a change from baseline.[1] Subjective symptoms, on the other hand, may be sensitive to poor insight by the patient or exaggeration by caregivers. Culture, education, gender, and occupation may all play a role in the level of awareness of and reaction to a patient's cognitive decline.[1]

Although there is no single, conclusive test to diagnose dementia, PCPs have several tools available for identifying symptoms and severity. For a patient at risk for dementia, rapid screening tests for cognitive impairment can determine if a more comprehensive evaluation is warranted.[1–3,5,13] Screening should not be restricted to patients 65 years and older. The 2015 Behavioral Risk Factor Surveillance System survey estimated that 12% of Americans age 45 years and older reported "subjective cognitive decline," one of the earliest signs of dementia.[2] Of those who reported it, only 44% consulted a health care professional about it.[2]

The following rapid screening tests are recommended by the American Academy of Family Physicians[14]:

- Verbal fluency test: naming as many animals as possible in 60 seconds
- Mini-Cognitive Assessment Instrument: 3-item recall combined with clock-drawing test
- Sweet 16: 3-item repetition and recall, 8-item orientation, and backward 5-digit span

More in-depth cognitive assessments include the Mini-Mental State Examination (MMSE) and the Montreal Cognitive Assessment (MoCA).[15–17] MMSE is a 30-question test that assesses cognitive function in the domains of orientation, attention, memory, language, and construction abilities.[15,17] MoCA is a 1-page assessment administered in 10 minutes and tests short-term memory, visuospatial abilities, attention, concentration, working memory, language, and orientation.[16] In patients with suspected dementia, it is important to evaluate specific cognitive deficits using a method to assess multiple domains, such as MMSE or MoCA.[1–4] Cognitive performance on these tests were shown to vary by age and education. High levels of education can result in false-negative examinations, whereas lower education levels can lead to false-positive results. Furthermore, age is an additional confounding factor that should be considered when establishing cutoff points for interpretation.[16,18,19]

The second criterion for functional decline applies only to the diagnoses of dementia or major NC, but not to MCI or minor NCD.[1–5] Functional decline is most often detected when taking the history from an informant, friend, or family member, although several easy scales can facilitate this process, and often if the impairment is mild, subjects themselves may be able to provide evidence for such decline. Caution should be noted when taking a history from an impaired person because anosognosia, or a loss of awareness of one's own disease processes, is often seen in even mild stages of MCI or dementia.[1,2,4] The Functional Assessment Questionnaire (FAQ) is a brief set of 10 questions for the informant that may help to tease out evidence for functional decline, and several other instruments like it are available for use in diagnosis.[1–5,14] In addition to an informant's functional assessment, several other tools are also available to help assess subjective decline in function. Objective tests of functional impairment have been developed but are not used commonly in the assessment of NCD, including both minor (MCI) and major (dementia) NCD.[1,2]

The third criterion for diagnosis includes evaluation of nondegenerative or medical causes for cognitive and or functional decline. This is a critical step in the evaluation process because there are currently no cures for any of the degenerative dementias, but treatments may be available for the many nondegenerative or medical causes for MCI or dementia.[1–5,20] The American Academy of Neurology practice parameter on the initial diagnosis and evaluation of dementia specifies routine laboratory work and brain imaging as critical componenst of the medical assessment.[3] Nondegenerative or medical cause(s) for such decline include metabolic dysregulation (eg, hyponatremia, hypo or hyperglycemia, uremia, and hyperammonemia), endocrine abnormalities (eg, hypothyroidism and hyperparathyroidism), nutritional deficiencies (eg, vitamin B_1 or vitamin B_{12} deficiencies), depression, delirium, medication-related adverse effects (eg, anticholinergic drugs), infections, poisoning, brain tumors, anoxia or hypoxia, stroke, cardiac and respiratory problems, and alcohol or substance abuse, among others.[21,22] Early recognition of abnormal cognitive decline should be an important trigger for medical investigations into the cause for such signs and symptoms.[5,7] The American Academy of Neurology practice parameter includes recommendations that assess the most prevalent of these alternative etiologies that may be responsible for the cognitive and or functional decline seen in a patient (**Table 2**).[3,20]

The fourth criterion includes screening for psychiatric disease as the root cause for the observed cognitive and or functional decline. Screening for depression is especially important and many tools are available to the clinician and their staff, including the Geriatric Depression Scale, which is available in both 15-item and 30-item forms and in multiple languages, that can be filled out by the patient prior to examination.[1–5,7] Other commonly used tools include the Neuropsychiatric Inventory, which

Table 2
Routine diagnostic work-up for nondegenerative or medical causes of cognitive and/or functional decline according to the American Academy of Neurology practice parameter on dementia[a]

Test	Recommendation
Complete blood cell count	Should test
Serum electrolytes	Should test
Glucose	Should test
SUN/creatinine	Should test
Vitamin B$_{12}$ level	Should test
Thyroid function tests	Should test
Liver function tests	Should test
RPR (syphilis screen)	Do not test unless high suspicion for exposure exists
Structural neuroimaging (noncontrast CT or MRI scan)	Should test
Volumetric structural analysis of CT or MRI scan	Do not test
Genetic testing	Do not test
PET (FDG, amyloid, or tau)	Do not test (although FDG PET is now approved by CMS for use in distinguishing AD from FTD as its only indication in the area of dementia)
SPECT	Do not test
CSF analysis	Do not test
14-3-3 for suspicion of CJD	Should test if suspicion for CJD is high

Abbreviations: ADS, Alzheimer disease; BUN, serum urea nitrogen; CJD, Creutzfeldt-Jakob disease; CMS, Centers for Medicare & Medicaid Services; FTD, frontotemporal dementia; RPR, rapid plasma reagin; SPECT, single-proton emission CT.

[a] The current American Academy of Neurology practice parameter was last updated in 2001, so may not have taken into consideration emerging evidence for the utility of some of the testing that is currently not recommended but has accumulated supporting evidence for use in the past 2 decades.

From Knopman DS, DeKosky ST, Cummings JL, et al. Practice parameter: diagnosis of dementia (an evidence-based review). Report of the Quality Standards Subcommittee of the American Academy of Neurology. Neurology 2001;56(9):1143–53; with permission.

requires a family member, friend, or informant but explores a wider array of dementia-related psychiatric comorbidities that may not only assist in diagnosis but also serve to identify meaningful symptoms that may be targets for therapeutic intervention.[1–5,7]

For persons with moderate to severe dementia, the Cornell Scale for depression screening is useful. The Cornell Scale focuses on a caregiver interview regarding the 19 items of the scale and a brief interview of the person with dementia.[23]

The Role of Biomarkers in the Current Diagnosis of Dementia

Over the past decade, several antemortem biomarkers have been developed to identify specific causes of dementia, including cerebrospinal fluid (CSF) biomarkers for Alzheimer disease, amyloid-PET imaging, fludeoxyglucose (FDG)-PET imaging, and volumetric MRI measures, all commercially available.[1–4,14] Other research tools include MRI measures, such as diffusion tensor imaging, arterial spin labeling, functional MRI, magnetic resonance spectroscopy, tau-PET imaging, and a host of blood and CSF-based biomarkers that remain experimental.[2–4] These biomarkers are traditionally not compensated for by third-party payers so remain out of reach of most persons under diagnostic evaluation unless they are engaged in active research studies using such measures. Currently, biomarkers' use beyond the standard work-up for dementia are not needed to establish diagnosis although a primary practitioner should realize that the diagnostic landscape is in flux and it is possible that such measures could become routine practice in the near future.[1-3]

Whatever the tools used, the approach should be the same, focusing on the 4 key aspects of the diagnosis, discussed previously. A suggested algorithm for patient assessment is shown in **Fig. 4**.

TREATMENT
General Management Principles

Dementia is a progressive disorder with cognitive impairments and behavioral changes that cause significant distress to patients and caregivers.[2] Patients display a wide range of symptoms that are expected to develop and change over time.[2,4] As such, treatment plans should be individualized, be multimodal, and include regular monitoring for the emergence, progression, or regression of symptoms. Behavioral, psychosocial, and pharmacologic interventions are often used in concert with one another, but it is best to implement changes one at a time to ensure that the effects of each intervention can be properly evaluated.[4,24]

Routine outpatient care requires regular follow-up visits with either a PCP or psychiatric specialist, and the interval between visits should be based on clinical needs. Even a patient with seemingly stable dementia should be seen at least every 3 to 6 months. Patients who present a particularly complex clinical picture or have frequent acute episodes may need to be seen weekly or monthly. Intensive outpatient treatment programs and even temporary hospitalization are also needed at times for patients with acute care needs. As dementia progresses and care needs

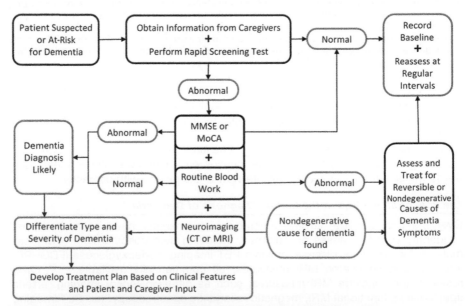

Fig. 4. Suggested algorithm for assessment of suspected dementia or MCI.

rise higher than can be afforded in the home environment, escalation to assisted living, personal care, or even skilled nursing facilities may be necessary as part of an ongoing care plan.[2]

Pharmacologic Treatment

There is, unfortunately, no cure at present for any of the degenerative causes of dementia.[2,4] The goal of pharmacotherapy in the dementia patient is to counter or delay the progression of symptoms, with all efforts focused on maximizing and maintaining patient safety and quality of life.[2,4] A small group of medications are approved by the Food and Drug Administration for cognitive impairment in dementia.[2,4] A host of other medications are often used to treat behavioral, psychiatric, sleep, and motor symptoms; however, the current practice parameters always recommend nonpharmacologic approaches as the first-line approach to symptom management.[2,4,25]

Medication initiation and titration in dementia should follow the general rule, "Start low and go slow." Elderly patients are likely to have decreased clearance due to impaired renal and hepatic function and often have numerous medications and coexisting conditions that can interfere with drug absorption and metabolism.[26] Additionally, dementia patients may struggle to express subjective experiences of benefit or adverse effects of treatment. Prescribers should initiate medications at low starting doses and increase doses in small increments, avoiding frequent medication changes and large dose adjustments.[24,26]

Four drugs are approved and available for the treatment of dementia: 3 cholinesterase inhibitors (donepezil, rivastigmine, and galantamine) and memantine, a noncompetitive N-methyl-D-aspartate receptor antagonist (NMDA).[2,4,24] **Table 3** provides important details for each of these medications. Trials of all 4 dementia drugs, however, show only modest clinical benefit in slowing or reversing cognitive decline. Evidence is either nonexistent or weak for their efficacy in other non-Alzheimer dementias, although some evidence exists supporting their use in vascular dementia and dementia with Lewy bodies.[2,4,24] Practitioners should ensure that patients and caregivers understand the limitations of pharmacotherapy and maintain realistic expectations for treatment.

Unlike the cholinesterase inhibitors, which are now approved for all stages of dementia, memantine remains approved for use in moderate to severe Alzheimer disease only. It remains uncertain if memantine is useful in early dementia or in prodromal disease states, such as MCI.[2,4,24] Memantine can be used alone or in combination with a cholinesterase inhibitor and is available in a fixed-dose combination with donepezil. Systematic reviews have shown small but statistically significant benefits to combination therapy in moderate to severe Alzheimer dementia, but the clinical significance of these effects is still unclear.[2,4,24]

In addition to treating cognitive decline in dementia, pharmacotherapy is often sought for the treatment of psychiatric and behavioral symptoms, such as agitation, aggression, psychosis, and sleep disturbances.[4,25] Antipsychotics, benzodiazepines, and other hypnotics, however, should be used cautiously and only after nonpharmacologic interventions have failed.[26,27]

All antipsychotics carry a black box warning about increased risk of mortality in elderly patients, and the clinical antipsychotic trials of intervention effectiveness – alzheimer's disease (CATIE-AD) demonstrated that the modest symptom benefit of antipsychotics in Alzheimer disease is offset by adverse effects, including further cognitive impairment.[2,4,26,27] If antipsychotics are needed to ensure the safety of a patient or caregiver, the lowest effective dose should be used, and agents with significant anticholinergic

Table 3
Drugs for the treatment of cognitive symptoms

Drug	Formulations	Food and Drug Administration Indication	Adverse Effects	Prescribing Considerations	Comments
Cholinesterase inhibitors					
Donepezil	Tablet, orally disintegrating tablet	Alzheimer dementia, mild to moderate and moderate to severe	Nausea/vomiting, muscle cramps, bradycardia, syncope, decreased appetite, increased stomach acid, vivid/disturbing dreams	Caution in patients with cardiac conduction problems or history of ulcer. May exacerbate asthma, COPD, or sleep disturbance	Cholinergic side effects tend to fade within 1 wk of initiation. GI side effects may be lessened with transdermal preparations
Rivastigmine	Capsule, transdermal patch	Alzheimer's dementia, mild to moderate Parkinson's dementia, mild to moderate			
Galantamine	Tablet, extended release capsule, solution	Alzheimer dementia, mild to moderate			
Noncompetitive NMDA receptor antagonist					
Memantine	Tablet, extended release capsule, solution	Alzheimer dementia, moderate to severe	Mild confusion, dizziness, headache, sedation, constipation	Dose adjust for impaired renal function	Typically well tolerated

Abbreviations: COPD, chronic obstructive pulmonary disease; FDA, food and drug administration; GI, gastro-intestinal.
Data from Refs.[2,4,17,20]

effects should be avoided. Use of antipsychotics in dementia patients should be reassessed frequently, and periodic attempts to withdraw or reduce the dose should be made.[2,4,25–27]

The benefits of benzodiazepines are even less apparent. Benzodiazepines may be considered on an as-needed basis for patients in whom anxiety is prominent or when sedation is needed for a particular medical or dental procedure. Benzodiazepines carry significant risk, however, of oversedation, delirium, and disinhibition, and may worsen behaviors that caregivers are trying to prevent.[24–27]

There is no single pharmacologic approach to treating sleep disturbances in dementia. Diphenhydramine and other over-the-counter sleep aids should be avoided due to their anticholinergic properties.[24,26,27] Anticholinergic medications in general should be avoided in patients with dementia because they have a high risk of inducing severe adverse effects on cognition and psychiatric symptoms, including increasing psychotic symptoms and agitation.[28,29] Patients treated for other neuropsychiatric conditions may benefit from the use of a sedating medication close to bedtime (eg, mirtazapine for depression or a second-generation antipsychotic, such as olanzapine or quetiapine, for psychosis). Some clinicians prefer to prescribe low doses of trazodone at bedtime or a small dose of zolpidem or zaleplon. Clonazepam is frequently used for the treatment of rapid eye movement sleep behavior disturbance that can be frequently seen in dementia with Lewy bodies and Parkinson dementia.[4] All these options, however, increase the risk of rebound insomnia, daytime sleepiness, falls, and worsening cognition. For this reason, sleep hygiene, treatment of exacerbating conditions, and discontinuation of medications that interfere with sleep should be optimized before pursuing pharmacologic treatment of sleep disturbances.[24,26] Several studies have demonstrated some benefit of safer sleep aids, such as melatonin, although a definitive benefit has yet to be proved.[4,24,26] These risks of most sleep aids, however, are not seen with melatonin, marking it as a safer alternative to conventional pharmaceutical sleep aids.

Pharmacologic Treatment of Behavioral and Psychiatric Symptoms of Dementia

Although cognitive decline is a primary symptom of dementia, neuropsychiatric and behavioral symptoms are often primary targets for symptomatic treatment. These symptoms are often best addressed by behavioral specialists who may provide in-depth psychotherapy or design behavioral or nonpharmacologic interventions to eliminate or reduce specific symptoms.[4,24,26]

Neuropsychiatric and behavioral symptoms tend to be particularly distressing to caregivers and family, who should be educated on techniques to mitigate symptoms and be reassured that behavioral symptoms can often be improved or eliminated with appropriate treatment.[2] The Alzheimer's Association Web site is a useful resource for your patients and their caregivers. The American Psychiatric Association *Practice Guideline for the Treatment of Patients with Alzheimer's Disease and Other Dementias* recommends educating family in the following basic principles of care[24]:

- Recognizing declines in capacity and adjusting expectations appropriately
- Bringing sudden declines in function and the emergence of new symptoms to professional attention
- Keeping requests and demands relatively simple
- Deferring requests if a patient becomes overly upset or angered
- Avoiding overly complex tasks that may lead to frustration
- Not confronting patients about their deficits

- Remaining calm, firm, and supportive and providing redirection if a patient becomes upset
- Being consistent and avoiding unnecessary change
- Providing frequent reminders, explanations, and orientation cues

PCPs likely also may find many of these basic principles helpful in the routine care of dementia patients.

Agitated dementia patients can often exhibit physical aggression, combativeness, and threatening behavior.[2,4] New or worsening agitation should be carefully assessed because it may be the result of an underlying medical condition (eg, urinary tract infection), untreated pain, or medication side effect. If medical intervention does not correct the agitated behavior, targeted behavioral interventions should be devised. If a behavior is dangerous to the patient or caregiver, however, and cannot be controlled, pharmacologic management, professional in-home care, or hospitalization must be considered.[2,4,24]

Social and Safety Interventions

As dementia progresses, it is important for PCPs to be acutely aware of the safety risks the disease imposes on patients and their caregivers.[2,4,25] Early conversations about the course of the disease can help patients and caregivers identify situations that put patients in danger and prepare everyone for decisions related to increased supervision and institutionalization.[30]

Typically, dementia patients should be cared for in the least restrictive environment that keeps them safe. As ability to perform ADLs declines, a patient's home environment should be assessed regularly. Practitioners should evaluate the patient's ability to take medications correctly and safely, the caregiver's ability to minimize and address wandering, and the sufficiency of a patient's resources and support from community resources.

Falls are a common problem for all elderly individuals and can lead to serious consequences. This problem is confounded by the development of comorbid Parkinsonism or motor neuron disease in degenerative dementias, such as dementia with Lewy bodies and frontotemporal dementia, or by focal neurologic deficits in those with cerebrovascular disease.[2,4] Environmental modifications, such as lowering beds, removing loose rugs, installing night lights, and rearranging furniture, can reduce fall risk. Additionally, gait disturbances should be addressed, and physical therapy may be appropriate for muscle strengthening and balance retraining.[24]

Even mild dementia impairs driving performance, and the risk of accidents increases with progression of the disease.[31] Regular discussions should be held among practitioners, patients, and caregivers to determine when a patient should stop driving. This decision should balance the risk of the patient's declining driving ability with the benefits of continued independence and access to community services.[31] The current American Academy of neurology practice parameter on driving and dementia provides several useful identifiers of impaired driving risk, including dementia beyond the mildest stage, a caregiver or informant's report of unsafe driving behaviors, and an MMSE score of less than or equal to 24, among others.[31] Practitioners should be aware that the regulations and legal requirements for assessing and reporting driving impairment vary by state (http://www.oregon.gov/ODOT/DMV/pages/at-risk_program_index.aspx), and each practitioner should be aware of local statutes and regulations regarding reporting requirements. The Automobile Association of America offers SeniorDriving.AAA.com that discusses the significance of driving assessment for older adults and also provides valuable resources.

SPECIAL ISSUES AND CONSIDERATIONS IN PRIMARY CARE SETTINGS

Patients with dementia often have significant comorbidities that complicate their care. Among Medicare beneficiaries age 65 and older, 26% of those with dementia have 5 or more chronic conditions, compared with only 3.8% of those without dementia.[2] For PCPs, the challenges faced by a patient with dementia affect treatment plans for all of a patient's disease states. Innovative care models, such as employing a professional to serve as a care manager, may be needed to ensure that plans are appropriate, coordinated, and relayed to a patient's caregivers.[2]

PCPs should carefully consider a patient's cognitive skills when explaining treatment plans and should provide all treatment information in a written form that can be taken home. Medication regimens should be simplified as much as possible, with schedules provided in an easy-to-follow format. Locked, timed dispensing devices are available for patients whose caregivers cannot be present for all medication administrations.

PCPs should ensure that treatments for other disease states do not exacerbate the dementia patient's condition.[2,24,27] For instance, in patients with dementia and type 2 diabetes mellitus, treatment goals should take into account the higher risk for hypoglycemic event that can further accentuate cognitive impairment and aggravate their health status.[32,33] Specifically, aggressive treatment goals of lowering of hemoglobin A_{1c} to address the potential for long-term harm induced by hyperglycemia might not be relevant for patients with dementia who are at higher risk from experiencing hypoglycemic episodes that can worsen their dementia symptoms.[34,35] In addition, each patient with dementia should receive optimal medical care that takes into account not only the standards of care but also the individual patient and caregiver preferences. PCPs can help establish individualized treatment goals to optimize health and function for the patient while considering patient and caregiver.[36] Given the frequency of polypharmacy in the elderly, a patient's full medication regimen should be reviewed regularly for drugs that may be adversely affecting cognitive function or placing the patient at increased risk for falls, delirium, or respiratory depression. Medications with anticholinergic effects or known to cause dizziness, sedation, or confusion should be avoided.[2,24,26,27] The prescriber should carefully weigh the risks and benefits of each medication and choose the lowest risk medication that appropriately treats the patient's condition. For example, in treating depression, selective serotonin reuptake inhibitors are preferred to the more sedating, anticholinergic tricyclic antidepressants.

Finally, PCPs should not ignore the mental and physical well-being of the caregiver, because this often has a direct effect on the care of the dementia patient.[2] Patients whose caregivers are exhausted, frustrated, or overwhelmed are at higher risk for abuse or neglect.[2,24] Providing the primary caregiver with resources for case management, support groups, respite care, and counseling can help improve the lives of both caregiver and patient.[2,24]

SUMMARY

Despite the fact that degenerative diseases remain incurable, they should be actively diagnosed and treated to maintain and or improve safety and quality of life for both patients and their immediate caregivers. Diagnostic criteria are constantly evolving, yet the core features remain stable.[4] The ability to recognize subtle cognitive decline and in many instances find a medically reversible or nondegenerative cause that can be remedied remains a major impetus for such diagnosis.[2,4,5,20] A rational understanding of the interplay between the development of dementia and the ongoing care of other chronic health conditions is critical for the development of appropriate treatment plans that ensure maximal benefit, reduce potential harm, and ensure that quality of life is maximized for aging patients. MCI and dementia deserve to be diagnosed and treated with the same rigor with which other chronic health conditions, such as diabetes, kidney failure, chronic obstructive pulmonary disease, hypertension, and all the other maladies of aging, are approached. Until potential cures are found for each of the degenerative dementias, these diseases will remain among the most common chronic health conditions affecting the elderly in society today, and primary care clinics will continue to serve a crucial role as the first line of defense in their recognition and treatment.[2]

REFERENCES

1. American Psychiatric Association. Diagnostic and statistical manual of mental disorders: DSM-V. Washington, DC: APA Press; 2013.
2. Alzheimer's Association. 2017 Alzheimer's disease facts and figures. Alzheimers Dement 2017;13(4):325–74.
3. Knopman DS, DeKosky ST, Cummings JL, et al. Practice parameter: diagnosis of dementia (an evidence-based review). Report of the Quality Standards Subcommittee of the American Academy of Neurology. Neurology 2001;56(9):1143–53.
4. Jicha GA, Carr SA. Conceptual evolution in Alzheimer's disease: implications for understanding the clinical phenotype of progressive neurodegenerative disease. J Alzheimers Dis 2010;19(1):253–72.
5. Winblad B, Palmer K, Kivipelto M, et al. Mild cognitive impairment–beyond controversies, towards a consensus: report of the international working group on mild cognitive impairment. J Intern Med 2004;256(3):240–6.
6. Petersen RC, Doody R, Kurz A, et al. Current concepts in mild cognitive impairment. Arch Neurol 2001;58(12):1985–92.
7. Petersen RC, Stevens JC, Ganguli M, et al. Practice parameter: early detection of dementia: mild cognitive impairment (an evidence-based review). Report of the Quality Standards Subcommittee of the American Academy of Neurology. Neurology 2001;56(9):1133–42.
8. Petersen RC, Roberts RO, Knopman DS, et al. Prevalence of mild cognitive impairment is higher in men. The Mayo Clinic study of aging. Neurology 2010; 75(10):889–97.
9. Roberts RO, Geda YE, Knopman DS, et al. The incidence of MCI differs by subtype and is higher in men: the Mayo Clinic study of aging. Neurology 2012;78(5): 342–51.
10. Nelson PT, Schmitt FA, Jicha GA, et al. Association between male gender and cortical Lewy body pathology in large autopsy series. J Neurol 2010;257(11): 1875–81.
11. Daviglus ML, Plassman BL, Pirzada A, et al. Risk factors and preventive interventions for Alzheimer disease: state of the science. Arch Neurol 2011;68(9): 1185–90.
12. Hurd MD, Martorell P, Langa KM. Monetary costs of dementia in the United States. N Engl J Med 2013;369(5):489–90.
13. Langa KM, Larson EB, Crimmins EM, et al. A comparison of the prevalence of dementia in the United States in 2000 and 2012. JAMA Intern Med 2017;177(1): 51–8.
14. Simmons BB, Hartmann B, Dejoseph D. Evaluation of suspected dementia. Am Fam Physician 2011;84(8):895–902.

15. Cockrell JR, Folstein MF. Mini-mental state examination (MMSE). Psychopharmacol Bull 1988;24(4):689–92.

16. Nasreddine ZS, Phillips NA, Bédirian V, et al. The montreal cognitive assessment, MoCA: a brief screening tool for mild cognitive impairment. J Am Geriatr Soc 2005;53(4):695–9.

17. Folstein MF, Folstein SE, McHugh PR. "Mini-mental state". A practical method for grading the cognitive state of patients for the clinician. J Psychiatr Res 1975; 12(3):189–98.

18. Crum RM, Anthony JC, Bassett SS, et al. Population-based norms for the mini-mental state examination by age and educational level. JAMA 1993;269(18): 2386–91.

19. Rossetti HC, Lacritz LH, Cullum CM, et al. Normative data for the montreal cognitive assessment (MoCA) in a population-based sample. Neurology 2011;77(13): 1272–5.

20. Jicha GA, Abner E, Schmitt FA, et al. Clinical features of mild cognitive impairment differ in the research and tertiary clinic settings. Dement Geriatr Cogn Disord 2008;26(2):187–92.

21. Alzheimer's Association. 2016 Alzheimer's disease facts and figures. Alzheimers Dement 2016;12(4):459–509.

22. Clarfield AM. The decreasing prevalence of reversible dementias: an updated meta-analysis. Arch Intern Med 2003;163(18):2219–29.

23. Alexopoulos GS, Abrams RC, Young RC, et al. Cornell scale for depression in dementia. Biol Psychiatry 1988;23(3):271–84.

24. Rabins PV. Practice guideline for the treatment of patients with Alzheimer's disease and other dementias, in Guideline watch. Washington, DC: APA Press; 2014.

25. Jicha GA, Nelson PT. Management of frontotemporal dementia: targeting symptom management in such a heterogeneous disease requires a wide range of therapeutic options. Neurodegener Dis Manag 2011;1(2):141–56.

26. Vrdoljak D, Borovac JA. Medication in the elderly - considerations and therapy prescription guidelines. Acta Med Acad 2015;44(2):159–68.

27. Counsell SR. 2015 updated AGS Beers Criteria offer guide for safer medication use among older adults. Geriatr Nurs 2015;36(6):488–9.

28. Fick DM, Cooper JW, Wade WE, et al. Updating the Beers criteria for potentially inappropriate medication use in older adults: results of a US consensus panel of experts. Arch Intern Med 2003;163(22):2716–24.

29. Sunderland T, Tariot PN, Cohen RM, et al. Anticholinergic sensitivity in patients with dementia of the Alzheimer type and age-matched controls. A dose-response study. Arch Gen Psychiatry 1987;44(5):418–26.

30. Jicha GA. Medical management of frontotemporal dementias: the importance of the caregiver in symptom assessment and guidance of treatment strategies. J Mol Neurosci 2011;45(3):713–23.

31. Iverson DJ, Gronseth GS, Reger MA, et al. Practice parameter update: evaluation and management of driving risk in dementia: report of the Quality Standards Subcommittee of the American Academy of Neurology. Neurology 2010;74(16): 1316–24.

32. Yaffe K, Falvey C, Hamilton N, et al. Diabetes, glucose control, and 9-year cognitive decline among older adults without dementia. Arch Neurol 2012;69(9): 1170–5.

33. Feil DG, Rajan M, Soroka O, et al. Risk of hypoglycemia in older veterans with dementia and cognitive impairment: implications for practice and policy. J Am Geriatr Soc 2011;59(12):2263–72.
34. Kirsh SR, Aron DC. Choosing targets for glycaemia, blood pressure and low-density lipoprotein cholesterol in elderly individuals with diabetes mellitus. Drugs Aging 2011;28(12):945–60.
35. Thorpe CT, Gellad WF, Good CB, et al. Tight glycemic control and use of hypoglycemic medications in older veterans with type 2 diabetes and comorbid dementia. Diabetes Care 2015;38(4):588–95.
36. Ibrahim JE, Anderson LJ, MacPhail A, et al. Chronic disease self-management support for persons with dementia, in a clinical setting. J Multidiscip Healthc 2017;10:49–58.

Evaluation of the Older Driver

Lucia Loredana Dattoma, MD

KEYWORDS

- Older driver • Older adult driver • Driving ability
- Clinical assessment of driving-related skills (CADReS) • Driving life expectancy

KEY POINTS

- The *Clinician's Guide to Assessing and Counseling Older Drivers*, 3rd Edition is published by the American Geriatrics Society in collaboration with the National Highway Traffic Safety Administration.
- Step I of the plan for the older driver safety screens for patients at risk includes the assessment of the physical, cognitive, driving ability, and medical conditions domains.
- Step II involves the clinical assessment of the following 4 domains: interview and history, vision screening, motor and sensory function, and cognitive testing.
- Step III allows for the clinician to identify, correct, and stabilize any underlying medical condition causing a functional deficit and, therefore, impairing the older adult's driving performance.
- Step IV is the final step in that the clinician uses the data collected in steps I to III to provide recommendations and devise an individualized plan.

INTRODUCTION

Older adults in the United States today are by far healthier and more active than ever before. Today the baby boomer generation is aging and is the most rapidly growing demographic. Currently in the United States 17% of the population and 46 million are aged 65 years or older, and approximately 79% of older adults aged 70 years and older have a driver's license. The number of older adult drivers 65 years of age and older is increasing rapidly as our older population increases. It is predicted that by 2050 there will be 2 times as many older adults, approximately 89 million, which will comprise 25% of all licensed drivers. However, most of the 89 million older adults will require transportation as they are outliving their ability to drive safely by an average of 7 to 10 years. According to a survey conducted in 2001 to 2003 by the Centers for Disease Control and Prevention, 75% of older adults aged 75 to 84 years and 70% of those aged 85 years and older were current drivers.[1]

No conflicts of interest to report.
Division of Geriatrics, Department of Medicine, UCLA School of David Geffen, 10945 LeConte Avenue # 2339, Los Angeles, CA 93065, USA
E-mail address: LDattoma@mednet.ucla.edu

Prim Care Clin Office Pract 44 (2017) 457–467
http://dx.doi.org/10.1016/j.pop.2017.05.003
0095-4543/17/© 2017 Elsevier Inc. All rights reserved.

primarycare.theclinics.com

Recently, older drivers have become front page news not only because they are an aging population but they are also involved in more fatal car incidents per miles driven than any other age group except teenagers. Motor vehicle accidents are the leading cause of injury-related deaths among adults aged 65 to 74 years and the second among those aged 75 to 84 years. In 2013, 5671 older adults were killed and 222,000 were injured in motor vehicle accidents.[2]

One thing that is evident in aging older drivers is that even though there may be signs of a moderate decline in mentation and psychomotor, ophthalmic, and auditory functions, many still drive safely. This fact is the case because most driving patterns are learned, embedded in long-term memory, and become second nature. In addition, older drivers tend to regulate their own driving with time. They drive shorter distances and fewer miles, and they drive minimally at night and seldom during rush hour.[1] Generally, driving performance may become impaired only after a significant loss of function occurs.

Driving is very important for older adults as it is critical to their independence and self-esteem. However, often older adults are forced to stop driving and as a result rely more on their families for transportation and accomplishing day-to-day tasks. This dynamic can lead to reduced social activities, and older adults lacking in transportation options often become depressed and isolated.

CLINICAL PREVENTION OF DRIVING DISABILITY

Clinical prevention strategies are a common core of knowledge for health professions in which individual- and population-oriented efforts provide prevention and health promotion. The clinical prevention strategy for driving disability is broken down into 3 categories: primary, secondary, and tertiary prevention. Each category is defined next.

Primary prevention assesses the older adult driver and intervenes to prevent the loss of driving ability. For example, visual deficit occurs because of worsening cataracts. The intervention is defined as primary prevention and consists of patients undergoing cataract excision. *Secondary prevention* addresses issues already affecting driving skills and attempts to restore those skills through treatment and rehabilitation. For example, osteoarthritis affects turning ability of the neck or the hand grip on the wheel. The intervention is defined as the secondary prevention, which consists of undergoing physical and/or occupational therapy and learning to effectively use the mirrors. *Tertiary prevention* identifies loss of driving skills for which there is no compensatory strategy; therefore, recommendations of alternatives should be made to prevent harm to the older adult and others when driving is no longer an option.[3]

ROLE OF THE HEALTH CARE PROVIDER

The *Clinician's Guide to Assessing and Counseling Older Drivers*, 3rd Edition is published by the American Geriatrics Society (AGS) in collaboration with the National Highway Traffic Safety Administration as a resource for health care providers involved in the care of older adults and reflects the interprofessional nature of the team caring for an older adult driver. The role of the clinician is very important to the safety and longevity of driving, and the points on how to do that are listed in **Box 1**.

The health care provider should start by making a plan for older driver safety[3] by breaking the assessment into 4 steps: (I) screening for risk by addressing issues or concerns, (II) conducting a clinical assessment, (III) undergoing an in-depth evaluation, and (IV) openly discussing the testing results and outcomes.[3]

Box 1
Role of the health care provider in maintaining driver safety and longevity

- Maximize older adults driving life expectancy to match their life span and activity levels
- Promote health and fitness to preserve skills
- Minimize injuries in a potential crash
- Prevent fatalities to the older adults and others sharing the road
- Work with other interprofessional team members in different settings of care
- Assist with transitioning to alternative transportation options when it is no longer possible to drive safely

Data from Sims RV, Owsley C, Allman RM, et al. A preliminary assessment of the medical and functional factors associated with vehicle crashes by older adults. J Am Geriatr Soc 1998;46(5):556.

STEP I: SCREENING AND OBSERVATION

A health care provider initiates the driver screening assessment by identifying patients who are at high risk of unsafe driving. However, it is important to keep in mind that identifying a person at risk does not automatically assume that the driver is unsafe now. In addition, screening will identify more people than actually need an intervention; but the overall goal is to catch at-risk drivers early in an effort to prevent disability and harm.

The clinician should take into account any medical condition of concern, including either a new diagnosis or change in condition, and any signs and symptoms of concern on review of symptoms. Questions regarding the physical, cognitive, and driving ability should be conducted in this step of the plan for older driving safety. A physical assessment includes looking into sensory deprivation comprising impaired vision, hearing, decrease sensation in the extremities, and impaired mobility. The cognitive assessment includes inattention or loss of insight regarding personal care, difficulty with way finding (eg, getting to or leaving the office), and impaired memory, language expression, or comprehension. In addition, difficulties or lack of insight related to managing medical encounters, such as missed appointments, repeated phones call for the same issues, or appearing on the wrong day are all red flags. See **Tables 1** and **2** for additional signs and symptoms and medical conditions of concerns.[4]

Table 1
Risk factors for assessing driving safety

Risk Factors	Signs and Symptoms
Physical	History of falls, impaired ambulation, vision/hearing impairment, functional impairment affecting use of pedals, decreased neck range of motion, slow responses to visual or auditory cues
Cognitive	Impairment in short-term memory, learning new information, way finding, attention, recognizing unsafe situations, and keeping names and dates accurately
Driving ability	Difficulty with making turns, turning the wheel, staying in the correct lane, judging space between cars or exits, hitting curbs during maneuvers, ignoring signs and/or lights, inappropriate speed, any incident and/or increased frequency of incidents

Adapted from American Geriatrics Society, Pomidor A, editors. Clinician's guide to assessing and counseling older drivers. 3rd edition. Washington, DC: National Highway Traffic Safety Administration; 2016. Report No. DOT HS 812 228; with permission.

Table 2
Medical conditions that can pose a great risk to safe driving

Acute Medical Events	Chronic Conditions
• Acute myocardial infarction	• Diseases/conditions affecting vision
• Cerebrovascular accident/traumatic brain injury	• Advanced renal disease: fatigue, weakness, and fluctuations in blood pressure
• Arrhythmias	• Cardiovascular disease
• Dizziness	• Neurologic
• Orthostatic hypotension	• Psychiatric disorders
• Syncope	• Diabetes mellitus
• Vertigo	• Hypothyroidism
• Surgery	• Musculoskeletal disability
• Seizure	• Respiratory disease on supplemental oxygen
• Delirium	• Cancer/chemotherapy treatment
• New sedating medications	• Chronic debility

Adapted from American Geriatrics Society, Pomidor A, editors. Clinician's guide to assessing and counseling older drivers. 3rd edition. Washington, DC: National Highway Traffic Safety Administration; 2016. Report No. DOT HS 812 228; with permission.

Screening for at-risk drivers should include questions directed at the patients and/ or loved ones regarding driving ability (**Fig. 1**). The following questions are a good start:

1. Is the older adult a current or former driver? Does the older adult want to continue driving? Or does the older adult have to drive?
2. How often and under what circumstances does he or she drive?
3. Were there any driving incidents or changes in the past 5 years?
4. Are there any driving concerns that either the older adult or caregiver may have?
5. Does the older adult feel comfortable and want to continue driving?

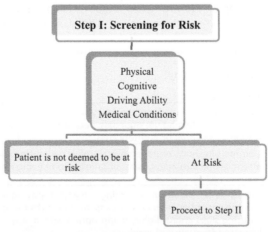

Fig. 1. Algorithm for step I (screening for risk). (*Data from* Marottoli R. The assessment of the older drivers. In: Hazzard WR, Blass JP, Halter JB, et al, editors. Principals of geriatric medicine and gerontology. 4th edition. McGraw-Hill: New York; 1999; p. 267–74. with permission.)

STEP II: CLINICAL ASSESSMENT

The second step in the plan for the older driver safety includes the Clinical Assessment of Driving-Related Skills (CADReS).[3,4] If patients are not deemed to be a safety driving risk, then this is an opportunity to discuss transportation options should patients need it and/or prepare for when the individual is required to quit driving. If patients are deemed to be at risk, the clinician should look further into identifying the impairment to build a plan of care exploring remediation and intervention by gathering data in domains associated with driving risk. This step is about assessing function, not age or diagnosis (**Fig. 2**).

Step II involves the clinical assessment of 4 domains:

- Interview and history: Assess whether patients currently drive (exposure, avoidance, self-limitations, accidents and citations, driving space).
- Vision screening: Test visual acuity and fields.
- Motor and sensory function: A history of falls has been associated with increased driving risk.
- Cognitive: Cognitive screening tests are controversial, but studies have suggested that these tests are useful in identifying patients at increased risk for unsafe driving. While assessing patients' cognition, it is important to keep in mind that cognitive impairment primarily with impaired attention, executive function, visual spatial ability, and information processing speed are the features most linked to impaired driving.

See **Table 3** for useful screening tools to assess each of the aforementioned domains.

The forms for each test and how to administer and score each screening tool are found online and in the *Clinician's Guide to Assessing and Counseling Older Drivers*.[3] One thing to remember is that not all screening tools have to be administered to assess the older driver. The clinician can decide which tools to use based on the patients' ability to pursue testing.

The Modified Driving Habits Questionnaire is broken down into 30 questions and 5 different categories, including a current driving history, exposure, avoidance, accidents and citations, and driving space. This questionnaire helps the clinician understand where patients are in regard to current driving and future planning. The value of the questionnaire for primary care clinicians is to identify functional measures that differentiate older adults who drive safely from those who do not.

Part of assessing patients' functional ability is finding out about their personal ability to care for themselves by assessing their activities of daily living (ADLs) and instrumental ADLs (IADLs). The ADLs include self-care tasks, such as feeding, toileting,

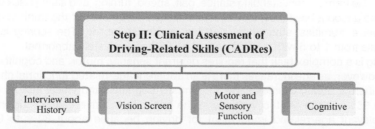

Fig. 2. Algorithm for step II (CADReS). (*Data from* Marottoli R. The assessment of the older drivers. In: Hazzard WR, Blass JP, Halter JB, et al, editors. Principals of geriatric medicine and gerontology. 4th edition. McGraw-Hill: New York; 1999; p. 267–74. with permission.)

Table 3	
Screening tools available for the assessment of each domain in step II	
Domain	**Screening Tools**
Interview and history	• Modified Driving Habits Questionnaire • Activities of Daily Living (ADLs) • Instrumental Activities of Daily Living (IADLs)
Vision screen	• Snellen chart • Ophthalmology consult may be necessary
Motor and sensory function	• Rapid Pace Walk and Range of Motion • Get up and Go Test
Cognitive	• Snellgrove Maze Task: www.snellgrovemazetask.com • Montreal Cognitive Assessment (MoCA): www.mocatest.org • Trail-Making Tests A/B: http://blog.hawaii.edu/dop/files/2011/08/trail-making-test.pdf • Clock drawing: www.nccdglobal.org/sites/default/files/content/clox.pdf

Adapted from American Geriatrics Society, Pomidor A, editors. Clinician's guide to assessing and counseling older drivers. 3rd edition. Washington, DC: National Highway Traffic Safety Administration; 2016. Report No. DOT HS 812 228; with permission.

dressing, bathing, incontinence, and transferring. The IADLs are more complex skills required to live independently, and those include proper use of the telephone, managing finances, handling transportation (driving or navigating public transportation), shopping, preparing meals, managing medications, laundry, and housekeeping. As a result of age-related declines in health, and physical and cognitive function, which leads to deterioration in ADLs and eventually IADLs, driving becomes more difficult for older adults. Many older adults eventually reduce or stop their driving activities, which may have adverse health consequences. Additionally, health problems are the most commonly cited reasons for driving cessation.[5]

A vision screen includes an in-office Snellen chart visual acuity assessment, and an ophthalmologist may assist with testing visual fields and managing vision changes. If hearing is of concern to patients, caregiver, or family member, a referral to an audiologist would be helpful for testing and hearing loss management.

Motor sensory ability can be tested using the Rapid Pace Walk or the Get Up and Go Test. Both will assess the bilateral lower extremity strength, range of motion, balance and endurance. The Rapid Pace Walk is a 10-ft path that patients must walk and then return back down the same path for a total 20-ft walk. The walk should be timed, and a score of 9 seconds or less is considered a normal test. The Get Up and Go test is similar to the Rapid Pace Walk in that it is a 10-ft walk but also assesses patients' sitting posture, rise from a chair, standing stance, gait, speed, turning, and sitting back down. It takes into account hesitancy, slowness, abnormal movements of the trunk and upper and lower extremities, staggering, shuffling, and/or stumbling. The scoring is based on a scale from 1 to 5 with 1 being normal and 5 being severely abnormal.

Driving is a complex task that requires different sensory, motor, and cognitive functions. However, as age increases there is an apparent age-related functional change in these different areas. Studies show that mostly cognition and visual factors explain 83% to 95% of age-related variance in the capacity to drive safely.[6] Vision is the most relevant age-related impairment for driving because about 80% to 90% of traffic-relevant information is taken in visually. Hearing is also strongly impaired because of normal aging but assumed to be less significant for traffic security. Driving ability and general mobility is influenced by age-related motor changes as muscle strength decreases and the speed of movement is reduced in addition to deterioration in motor coordination and dexterity.[6] Lastly, age-related cognitive changes can reflect a deterioration in fluid intelligence; such functions are important for the solution of problems and coping with unexpected traffic situations.[7]

The cognition is evaluated by any or all of the following assessment tools: the Maze test, the Montreal Cognitive Assessment, the Trail-Making Tests A/B, and the clock-drawing test. These tests are merely screening tools and are not diagnostic tests. However, they do help to assess visuospatial ability, executive function, attention and psychomotor coordination, language, and memory. A positive screening test will require referral to a dementia specialist and may preclude patients from driving until a diagnosis is established.

STEP III: EVALUATION OF THE SCREENING AND CLINICAL ASSESSMENT OF DRIVING-RELATED SKILLS

Step III is the overall evaluation of the screening and CADReS assessment.[8] In this step the clinician's role is to identify, correct, or stabilize any underlying medical cause of the patients' functional deficits that may impair their driving performance. Together the clinician, patients, and families will address any area identified to be at risk in the CADReS assessment process. Additionally, a diagnostic evaluation, medication adjustment, and specialty referral, Including ophthalmology, cardiology, neurology, psychiatry, orthopedics, physical and occupation therapy, and/or speech therapy, may be necessary. When the patients' acute and/or chronic conditions have been optimized as much as possible, the clinician may consider a referral to an occupational therapy/driving rehabilitation specialist to optimize functional benefit (**Fig. 3**[8]).

The driving rehabilitation specialty evaluation offers several services, including educational programs, that often proves beneficial in the older driver that takes advantage of such services. These services are as follows:

- Driving refresher courses
- Driving school tests of driving skills
- The standardized road test at the licensing agency

The trained driving rehabilitation and safety programs also provide the comprehensive driving evaluation, which consists of clinical assessments of vision, physical

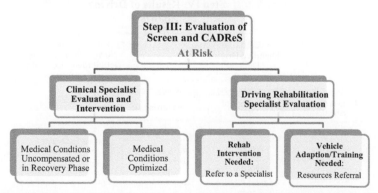

Fig. 3. Algorithm for step III (evaluation of screen and CADReS). (*Data from* Marottoli R. The assessment of the older drivers. In: Hazzard WR, Blass JP, Halter JB, et al, editors. Principals of geriatric medicine and gerontology. 4th edition. McGraw-Hill: New York; 1999; p. 267–74. with permission.)

capabilities, and cognition in even greater depth that the CADReS screen. These trained specialists working for comprehensive driving evaluation programs help clinicians identify strengths and concerns, explore solutions and generates an individualized plan.

Driver rehabilitation evaluation and training programs are available and often found at state.gov or department of motor vehicles (DMV) sites online by simply searching online for *driver's rehabilitation programs*. Here are a few examples:

Michigan State
New York State

STEP IV: DISCUSSION OF THE RESULTS OF A COMPREHENSIVE DRIVING EVALUATION

The overall results of the driving rehabilitation are to provide patients with recommendations and devise an individualized plan.[8] This process brings us to step IV in which the clinician consolidates the data collected in steps I to III and uses it to do the following:

1. Strategize options and empower patients with knowledge and lessons
2. Work on adaption skills and compensation
3. Provide information regarding equipment and vehicle modification[8]

If driving is the patients' ultimate goal, then options should be explored to make that possible. If there are no options suitable to allow patients to drive safely, then the driver should be assured that all options were explored. At this point the plan will involve cessation strategies and continued mobility as a pedestrian and/or encouraging transit use.[9] The aforementioned algorithms allow the clinician to explore options, offer hope, and equip themselves with data when preparing to deliver recommendations to patients. Although the original question may have been about driving, the outcome must address safe mobility with continued community access and isolation prevention (**Fig. 4**).

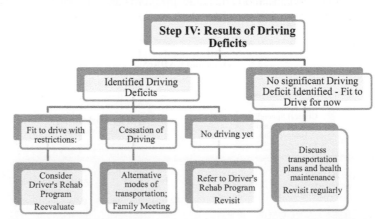

Fig. 4. Algorithm for step IV (results of driving deficits). (*Adapted from* Marottoli R. The assessment of the older drivers. In: Hazzard WR, Blass JP, Halter JB, et al, editors. Principals of geriatric medicine and gerontology. 4th edition. McGraw-Hill: New York; 1999; with permission.)

AGE-RELATED CHANGES THAT AFFECT DRIVING

The 3 most common age-related changes that occur in the older adult include changes in vision, hearing, psychomotor function, and cognitive status. In addition, older adults may have a range of mild to severe medical conditions that can affect functional performance and in turn affect driving performance. Some functional deficits have been identified as positive predictors of motor vehicle accidents and adverse driving incidents in the older adult population. These predictors are as follows:

1. Recent fall history as far back as in the last 1 to 2 years
2. Visual and cognitive deficits
3. A prior history of a motor vehicle accident and/or an adverse driving incident
4. The current use of medications (chronic, acute, or recent changes) including tricyclic antidepressants, opioids, antihistamines, and benzodiazepines[10]

The older adult population comprises about one-sixth of the US population, however, receive about one-third of all prescription drugs. It is estimated that the average older adult receives between 16 and 20 prescriptions drugs per year. This number does not include any over-the-counter or herbal supplements and/or alcohol use that patients may be adding to the regimen. It is important to counsel patients and take into account the physiologic changes associated with aging, which can affect drug absorption, distribution, and elimination. In addition, consider the adverse effects of all medications taken and assess for multiple drug interaction and whether all of the drugs being taken are absolutely necessary. Lastly, the physiologic changes of aging, such as decreased lean body mass and increased adipose tissue, can make alcohol a potent drug, especially when mixed in with other medically necessary medications a significant risk for the older driver.[11]

Mobility issues in the older adult that can impact driving include changes in muscle strength and flexibility, particularly of the neck, shoulder, and wrists, which limit reaction time and impact the ability to drive. Grip strength decreases; limitations in neck, shoulder, and wrist movement can reduce the field of vision in traffic situations as well as the ability to control and turn the steering wheel. Physical therapy and adaptive equipment, such as power assistive devices and special mirrors, can enhance driving ability and safety.

Once the clinician feels that patients may be unsafe to drive but patients or their families are not able to recognize the patients' limitations or patients refuse your assessment of their driving, it would be best to obtain an objective assessment. There are several resources in the community to further evaluate patients' driving abilities, including an on-the-road driving evaluation. Some resources to assess driving or to provide driving rehabilitation are the American Association of Retired Persons, which has an active older drivers program called 55 Alive and provides classes on driver safety. The Alzheimer's Association and the AGS are also good resources of information for clinicians, patients, and families.

What if your patients should stop driving, have gone through third-party assessment, but refuse to stop driving? (Coach families to hide the car, hide the keys, and disable the car.)

What if your patients lack decision-making capacity?

Know your state's reporting laws: Can or must physicians report to the DMV older patients at risk? Sometimes revoking the license will not stop a person from driving.

Be sure to offer alternatives to driving and refer patients to their Area Agency on Aging (AAA). The AAAs were established in 1973 under the Older Americans Act to respond to the needs of persons older than 60 years. They help older adults find services to help them age in place in their homes and communities. The AAAs have federal and state funding and social work professionals as well as networks of service providers to help older adults in the community. Read more about AAAs at n4a.org.

SUMMARY

With the silver tsunami among us and the advancement of medicine, the older adult population is increasing and remains healthier and more independent than ever. This circumstance has led to a longer driving life expectancy. However, although in the last 10 years, motor vehicle accident fatality has decreased overall, those accidents involving the older driver has actually increased overall. Therefore, driver safety discussions should begin early in the relationship established between the older adult and the clinician.

The role of the clinician is to begin by screening patients and discuss options for transportation when driving is no longer possible. If the screening assessment is positive, patients may benefit from referral to a specialist to assist with maintaining driving longevity. Remaining sincere and clear about the assessment, options, and recommendations is important throughout the clinical process.

The health care provider together with the cooperation of patients conducts a plan for the older driver safety. The plan includes 4 steps: (1) screening for risk by addressing issues or concerns, (2) conducting a clinical assessment, (3) undergoing an in-depth evaluation, and (4) discussing the test results and providing options. Once patients are deemed fit or unfit to drive right now, there are many resources that assist both the clinician and patients in attempting to maintain a healthy and safe driving life span. If continuing to drive is no longer an option, then together the patients and clinician will seek out alternatives for transportation and navigating the community. An interprofessional team is available to help both the clinician and patients seek the appropriate resources.

RESOURCES

1. GeriatricsCareOnline, http://geriatricscareonline.org
2. National Highway Traffic Safety Administration, http://www.nhtsa.gov/Driving+Safety/Older+Drivers
3. Association for Driver Rehabilitation Specialists, http://aded.site-ym.com/?page=725
4. NIH SeniorHealth, http://nihseniorhealth.gov/olderdrivers/howagingaffectsdriving/01.html
5. American Occupational Therapy Association, http://www.aota.org/Practice/Productive-Aging/Driving.aspx
6. Administration for Community Living, http://www.acl.gov/Get_Help/Help_Older_Adults/Index.aspx

REFERENCES

1. Betz ME, Lowenstein SR. Driving patterns of older adults: results from the second injury control and risk survey. J Am Geriatr Soc 2010;58:1931.
2. AAA. Roadwise review: a tool to help seniors drive safely longer. 2004.
3. American Geriatrics Society, Pomidor A, editors. Clinician's guide to assessing and counseling older drivers. 3rd edition. Washington, DC: National Highway Traffic Safety Administration; 2016. Report No. DOT HS 812 228.

4. Koepsell TD, Wolf ME, McCloskey L, et al. Medical conditions and motor vehicle collision injuries in older adults. J Am Geriatr Soc 1994;42(7):695.
5. Chihuru S, Mielenz TJ, DiMaggio CJ, et al. Driving cessation and health outcomes in older adults. J Am Geriatr Soc 2016;64(2):332–41.
6. Karthaus M, Falkenstein M. Functional changes and driving performance in older drivers: assessment and interventions. Geriatrics 2016;1:12.
7. Green KA, McGwin G, Owsley C. Associations between visual, hearing and dual sensory impairments and history of motor vehicle collision involvement of older drivers. J Am Geriatr Soc 2013;61(2):252–7.
8. Marottoli R. The assessment of the older drivers. In: Hazzard WR, Blass JP, Halter JB, et al, editors. Principals of geriatric medicine and gerontology. 4th edition. New York: McGraw-Hill; 1999. p. 267–74.
9. Betz ME, Jones VC, Lowenstein SR. Physicians and advanced planning for driving retirement. Am J Med 2014;127:689.
10. Ladden MD. Approach to the evaluation of the older drivers. UpToDate; 2015.
11. Hemmelgarn B, Suissa S, Huang A, et al. Benzodiazepine use and the risk of motor vehicle crash in the elderly. JAMA 1997;278:27.

The Older Adult with Diabetes and The Busy Clinicians

Rangaraj Gopalraj, MD, PhD

KEYWORDS

- Diabetes • Older adult • Geriatrics • Frailty • Life expectancy

KEY POINTS

- Older adults are more prone to diabetic complications and hypoglycemia.
- Target hemoglobin A1c level needs to be more relaxed for frail older adults.
- Lifestyle interventions are more effective in older adults.
- Geriatric syndromes adversely affect diabetes care.
- A team approach is vital.

OVERVIEW

Diabetes is a common problem in older adults (defined as >65 years of age). About 1 in 4 older adults, or more than 11 million individuals, in the United States who are 65 years of age and older are affected. Fueled in part by the obesity epidemic, this number is projected to double in the next 20 years and quadruple by 2050.[1,2] Diabetes takes a big toll on patients and families. Diabetes and its complications lead to higher mortality and nursing home placements in older adults. After adjusting for age and sex differences, patients with diabetes spend 2.3 times more for their medical care compared with those without diabetes.[3] This article focuses on how to approach older diabetics in terms of patient selection, hemoglobin A1c (A1c) goal setting, and being aware of the interplay between geriatric syndromes that can negatively affect these patients.

PATHOPHYSIOLOGY

Although increasing numbers of patients with type 1 diabetes live to be older, they comprise a minority of older adults with diabetes. More than 90% of diabetes in older adults is type 2, which is caused by insulin deficiency. Increasing age can adversely affect pancreatic islet function and islet cell proliferative capacity directly (**Fig. 1**). Older adults are also more susceptible to increased fat deposition, low muscle

Department of Family & Geriatric Medicine, University of Louisville, 1941 Bishop Lane, Suite 900, Louisville, KY 40218, USA
E-mail address: rkgopa01@louisville.edu

Prim Care Clin Office Pract 44 (2017) 469–479
http://dx.doi.org/10.1016/j.pop.2017.04.011
0095-4543/17/© 2017 Elsevier Inc. All rights reserved.

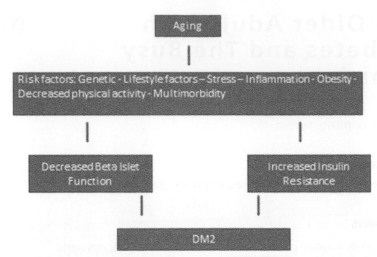

Fig. 1. Pathophysiology of diabetes in older adults. DM2, diabetes mellitus type 2.

mass, and physical inactivity. These factors can indirectly increase insulin resistance as well as decrease beta islet function.[4] This heightened susceptibility is one of the reasons why older adults respond disproportionately better with lifestyle interventions.[5]

SCREENING AND DIAGNOSIS

Given the high prevalence of diabetes in older adults, screening is recommended every 1 to 3 years in all adults starting from age 45 years. Identifying diabetes early could decrease the incidence of complications in older adults. It is ideal that the screened individuals have a long enough life expectancy to benefit from interventions. According to the American Diabetes Association in the absence of classic symptoms of hyperglycemia or hyperglycemic crisis coupled with a random plasma glucose level of ≥200 mg/dL, the following three measures such as a fasting plasma glucose level of ≥126 mg/dL, 2 hour oral glucose tolerance test ≥200 mg/dL, or an A1C level of ≥6.5% must be demonstrated on two separate occasions to confirm the diagnosis.

Postprandial hyperglycemia is a prominent characteristic in older adults.[6,7] Therefore when other criteria are relied on, like fasting plasma glucose or A1c level, up to one-third of the cases could be missed in older adults.[8] Medicare does not cover A1c for screening purposes unless other risk factors, such as family history or hyperglycemia, are present.

DIABETIC COMPLICATIONS IN SPECIFIC SUBPOPULATIONS OF OLDER ADULTS

Older adults with diabetes can be divided into 2 distinct subpopulations based on the age at onset. Some are diagnosed with diabetes early in life, such as in middle age, leading to long-standing diabetes, versus being incidentally found after they turn 65 years old. These two distinct subpopulations show differing demographics and clinical characteristics (**Table 1**).[9] The older onset of diabetes is seen more commonly in non-Hispanic white people; they tend to have lower mean A1c levels and less likely to be using insulin. The duration of diabetes seems to correlate with certain microvascular complications. For instance, retinopathy occurs more frequently in long-standing diabetes, and it increases progressively with increasing duration of diabetes. Poor

Table 1
Two broad subgroups of the older adult with diabetes

Age of Onset of Diabetes	Middle Age	Older Age
Age at Diagnosis (y)	<65	>65
More common in	—	Non-Hispanic Whites
Mean A1c level	Higher	Lower
Insulin use	Higher	Lower
Retinopathy	More common	Less common
Cardiovascular disease	About same	About same
Peripheral neuropathy	About same	About same

vision can affect compliance with medications, driving ability and independence. An annual eye examination with an ophthalmologist is recommended. Urinary microalbumin screening should be done annually to evaluate for nephropathy. Once identified, it may not be helpful to continue testing annually. Instead, if there are no contraindications, start angiotensin-converting enzyme inhibitor treatment for microalbuminuria. Peripheral neuropathy of the feet is common in older diabetics. Patients should proactively check their feet for any lesions or sores to prevent or identify problems early. Providers should assess patients' ability to visualize and reach their feet. Monofilament testing should be done annually and a podiatry consult can be helpful in the proper care of the feet.

HEMOGLOBIN A1C GOALS

A1c is a marker of glycemic control and has also emerged as a quality indicator. Tight glycemic control in younger and middle-aged adults is beneficial to health.

Reducing A1c level to less than or around 7.0% has been shown to reduce:

- Microvascular complications
- Macrovascular disease (if implemented soon after diagnosis)

However, in older adults, A1c levels of less than 6% have been shown to be harmful in increasing risk for dementia.[10] Even a more relaxed goal of less than 8% in frail older individuals was shown to cause adverse outcomes with troublesome hypoglycemia.[11] Therefore, instead of reflexively striving for a goal A1c of less than 7%, clinicians need to start by considering the patient characteristics first (**Fig. 2**).

Older adults are heterogeneous. They can range from being healthy and active in the community to having numerous comorbidities and being bed-bound in a nursing home. It is imperative that treatment goals are individualized (**Fig. 3**). The current recommendations from the American Geriatrics Society (AGS) and the American Diabetes Association (ADA) are:

- An A1c goal of less than 7.5% should be considered in medication-treated robust older patients.
- An A1c goal less than or equal to 8.0% should be considered in medication-treated frail older adults with medical and functional comorbidities and in those whose life expectancy is less than 10 years.
- Individualized goals for the very old may be even higher (A1c level <8.5%) and should include efforts to preserve quality of life and avoid hypoglycemia and related complications.

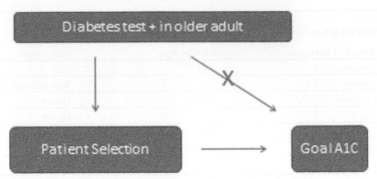

Fig. 2. Evaluate patient characteristics before setting goal A1c level.

The clinical guidelines are available at http://www.ndei.org/ADA-AGS-diabetes-older-adults-2012.aspx.html.

Targets need to be individualized based on several factors (**Table 2**), such as:

- Age/life expectancy
- Comorbid conditions
- Diabetes duration
- Concern for hypoglycemia

Lifestyle modification of 7% weight loss and 150 minutes of physical activity per week decreased the incidence of diabetes by 58%, and was found to be twice as effective as metformin at 850 mg 2 times a day compared with placebo in the Diabetes Prevention Program Study of at-risk individuals, which included 20% of subjects older than 60 years.[5] A 10-year follow-up study showed that older adults continued to

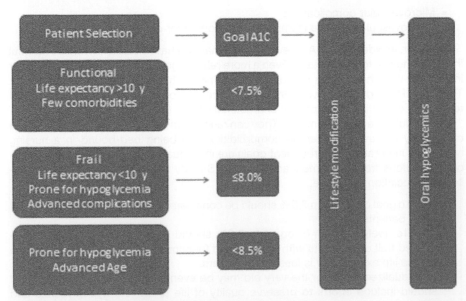

Fig. 3. Informed patient selection leads to appropriate goal A1c.

Table 2
Factors to consider in setting less or more stringent hemoglobin A1c targets

Target A1c	More Stringent	Less Stringent
Diabetes duration	Short	Long
Life expectancy	Long	Limited
Complications	Not yet developed	Advance microvascular or macrovascular
Comorbidities	Minimal	Extensive
Hypoglycemia	None	Severe

benefit from lifestyle interventions with less urinary incontinence and better quality-of-life scores.[12–14]

Older diabetics are often excluded from clinical studies, which can hamper evidence-based treatments for this vulnerable population. This tendency is especially true for individuals more than 75 years of age or in poor health. The UK Prospective Diabetes Study, which excluded adults 65 years of age and older at enrollment, showed the benefits of glycemic control in decreasing microvascular complications, which persisted into the poststudy follow-up period.[15–17] Subsequent studies, such as the Action to Control Cardiovascular Risk in Diabetes (ACCORD) trial, the Action in Diabetes and Vascular Disease: Preterax and Diamicron MR Controlled Evaluation (ADVANCE) trial, and the Veterans Affairs Diabetes Trial (VADT) were designed to examine the role of glycemic control in preventing cardiovascular disease events in middle-aged and older adults. The study subjects were 60 years old on average, with 8-year to 11-year histories of diabetes, and some even had prior cardiovascular events. In the most intensive therapy arm the goal was to decrease A1c level to less than 6% or less than 6.5%. Surprisingly, all 3 studies failed to show improvements in their primary outcome of reduced cardiovascular mortality with intensive glycemic control (**Table 3**). The ACCORD trial noted excessive deaths in the intensive glucose control arm, leading to its early termination at 3 years. The primary combined outcome of myocardial infarction, stroke, and cardiovascular death was not significantly reduced.[18] The ADVANCE trial did not report excessive deaths caused by glycemic control over a 5-year follow-up period; however, no significant cardiovascular benefits were shown either; it did show improved nephropathy.[19] Over 5 years the VADT showed no improvement in the rates of major cardiovascular events, death, or microvascular complications with the exception of progression of albuminuria with intensive glycemic therapy.[20] Intensive glycemic control was harmful in older individuals with longer-standing diabetes of 20 years or more in the VADT.[21]

Table 3
Major trials with older adults with diabetes

Trials	Primary Outcome of Decreased Cardiovascular Mortality	Notable Findings
ACCORD	Not demonstrated	Excessive deaths in intensive therapy arm leading to termination in 3 y
ADVANCE	Not demonstrated	Improved nephropathy
VADT	Not demonstrated	Intensive glycemic control was harmful in individuals with diabetes for ≥20 y

MANAGING COMORBIDITIES AND VASCULAR RISK FACTORS IN OLDER ADULTS WITH DIABETES

Older adults with diabetes have the highest rates of major lower-extremity amputation, myocardial infarction, visual impairment, and end-stage renal disease.[22] Diabetics more than 75 years of age have higher rates for most complications from the disease or its management. For instance, they visit emergency departments for hypoglycemia at twice the rate compared with younger adults.[23] Coexisting illnesses such as essential hypertension can accentuate insulin resistance[24] Hence, treating cardiovascular risk factors is beneficial for patients with a long life span. However, the ACCORD trial also cautions that intensive glycemic control in frail older adults can increase both total and cardiovascular disease mortality.[18]

A review of the pharmacologic treatment of hypoglycemia is beyond the scope of this article but is extensively discussed in other articles.[25,26] The salient features of oral agents that are commonly available in the United States are presented in **Table 4**.

INTERPLAY BETWEEN DIABETES AND GERIATRIC SYNDROMES

Diabetes increases the risk of many geriatric syndromes, which in turn negatively affects the management and outcomes of diabetes in older adults (**Fig. 4**). Diabetes is often part of a multimorbid phenotype. It coexists with obesity, low physical activity, poor diet, frailty, and insulin resistance. Diabetic individuals have been shown to have executive dysfunction and cognitive impairment.[27] Coexisting diabetes and cognitive impairment can lead to lower brain volume and accelerated cognitive dysfunction.[28] In earlier stages, cognitive impairment is harder to detect unless providers are specifically screening for this problem. Patients may have difficulty complying with treatment plans, may become more prone to hypoglycemia, or may have unexplained worsening of A1c level. Screening for cognitive impairment in this patient population is especially important. This screening can be achieved with a specific instrument that can be rapidly administered in the office, such as Mini-Cog.[29,30] This test consists of a 3-item recall and a standardized clock drawing with specific instructions on scoring. If positive, the patient can then be referred to a specialist such as a geriatrician or neurologist.

Depression is twice as common in diabetes.[31] Depressed diabetic patients may have worse glycemic control and complications such as coronary heart disease.[32] It is imperative to use a screening tool such as a Geriatric Depression Scale to identify and treat depression to improve outcomes.

Polypharmacy is common in managing the multiple comorbidities associated with diabetes.[33,34] Diabetic patients are twice as likely to have medication errors.[35] Clinicians need to be vigilant about drug interactions and side effects to avoid perpetuating a vicious cycle of treating side effects with additional medications.

The benefits of improved glycemic control in reducing complications, which can ultimately decrease falls risk, has to be weighed against the increased falls risk with intensive insulin therapy. Falls risk is increased in older adults because of multiple factors such as neuropathy, sarcopenia, frailty, sensory loss, polypharmacy, and hypoglycemia.[36] However, intensive glycemic control of HgbA1c levels less than 6% with insulin was associated with higher risk of falls.[37]

Urinary incontinence is more common in older diabetic women.[38] This incontinence could be related to urinary tract infections, autonomic neuropathy, or polyuria caused by hyperglycemia. This condition can affect quality of life.

Table 4
Oral medications for diabetes

Medications	Positives	Negatives
Biguanide • Metformin	Low risk of hypoglycemia No weight gain Long clinical experience Could decrease microvascular and macrovascular events	Stop if GFR is <30 Stop if ill or hospitalized GI adverse effects (common) Lactic acidosis (rare)
Sulfonylureas • Glipizide • Glyburide • Glimepiride	Low cost Long clinical experience Decreased microvascular events	Weight gain Hypoglycemia especially in long-acting agents (glyburide) Skin rash
Thiazolidinones • Pioglitazone	Minimal hypoglycemia Increased HDL level Decrease triglyceride level	Weight gain Heart failure Bone fractures
Meglitinides • Repaglinide • Nateglinide	Could be given before meals	Hypoglycemia Frequent dosing Weight gain
DPP-4 inhibitors • Sitagliptin • Saxagliptin • Linagliptin • Alogliptin	Once-daily dosing Well tolerated	Urticaria/angioedema Heart failure Pancreatitis Expensive
GLP-1 receptor agonists • Exenatide • Liraglutide • Dulaglutide • Albiglutide	Minimal hypoglycemia Weight reduction Decreased postprandial glycemic excursions	GI adverse effects Increased heart rate Thyroid tumors and pancreatitis in animal models
αGlucosidase inhibitors • Acarbose • Miglitol	Minimal hypoglycemia Decreased postprandial glycemic excursions	Flatulence Abdominal discomfort Frequent dosing Contraindicated in cirrhosis
Bile acid sequestrant • Colesevelam	Minimal hypoglycemia Decreased LDL level	Constipation Increased triglyceride level Expensive
Dopamine-2 agonist • Bromocriptine	Minimal hypoglycemia	Orthostatic hypotension, psychosis, nausea, headache Expensive
Amylinlike • Pramlintide	Weight reduction Decreased postprandial glycemic excursions	GI adverse effects Frequent dosing Expensive Potentiates hypoglycemia with insulin
SGLT-2 inhibitors • Canagliflozin • Empagliflozin • Dapagliflozin	Minimal hypoglycemia Weight reduction Once-daily dosing Reduces blood pressure	CI in chronic kidney disease Genitourinary infections Polyuria Orthostatic hypotension

Abbreviations: CI, contraindicated; DPP-4, dipeptidyl peptidase-4; GFR, glomerular filtration rate; GI, gastrointestinal; GLP-1, glucagonlike peptide-1; HDL, high-density lipoprotein; LDL, low-density lipoprotein; SGLT-2, sodium-glucose cotransporter-2.

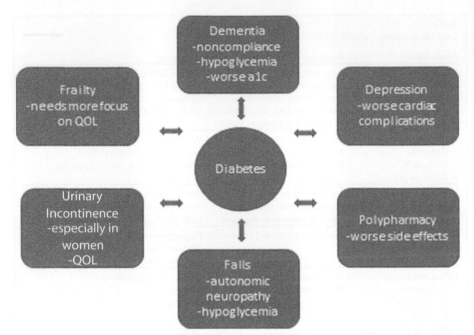

Fig. 4. Geriatric syndromes can affect care of the older adult with diabetes. QOL, quality of life.

Frailty in older adults is associated with metabolic syndrome, insulin resistance, and increased mortality.[39,40] Complex frail older adults are known to be at high risk for adverse outcomes with tight glycemic control. However, research shows that nearly half of these patients are still overtreated.[41]

SUMMARY

It takes a multidisciplinary effort to care for older adults with diabetes. A capable team that includes nursing staff, medicine and surgery subspecialists, social workers, pharmacists, mental health professionals, nutritionists, podiatrists, and physical and occupational therapists is vital. Busy primary care providers are in the frontlines and see the bulk of older adults with diabetes. Being aware of the heterogeneity of older adults, choosing an appropriately relaxed A1c goal, and capably leading a diverse care team can help provide quality care for patients and families struggling with diabetes and its aftermath.

REFERENCES

1. Boyle JP, Thompson TJ, Gregg EW, et al. Projection of the year 2050 burden of diabetes in the US adult population: dynamic modeling of incidence, mortality, and prediabetes prevalence. Popul Health Metr 2010;8:29.

2. Narayan KM, Boyle JP, Geiss LS, et al. Impact of recent increase in incidence on future diabetes burden: U.S., 2005-2050. Diabetes Care 2006;29(9):2114–6.

3. American Diabetes Association. Economic costs of diabetes in the U.S. in 2012. Diabetes Care 2013;36(4):1033–46.

4. Amati F, Dube JJ, Coen PM, et al. Physical inactivity and obesity underlie the in-sulin resistance of aging. Diabetes Care 2009;32(8):1547–9.
5. Knowler WC, Barrett-Connor E, Fowler SE, et al. Reduction in the incidence of type 2 diabetes with lifestyle intervention or metformin. N Engl J Med 2002; 346(6):393–403.
6. Chang AM, Halter JB. Aging and insulin secretion. Am J Physiol Endocrinol Metab 2003;284(1):E7–12.
7. Szoke E, Shrayyef MZ, Messing S, et al. Effect of aging on glucose homeostasis: accelerated deterioration of beta-cell function in individuals with impaired glucose tolerance. Diabetes Care 2008;31(3):539–43.
8. US Centers for Disease Control and Prevention. National diabetes statistics report: estimates of diabetes and its burden in the United States. 2014.
9. Selvin E, Coresh J, Brancati FL. The burden and treatment of diabetes in elderly individuals in the U.S. Diabetes Care 2006;29(11):2415–9.
10. Morita T, Okuno T, Himeno T, et al. Glycemic control and disability-free survival in hypoglycemic agent-treated community-dwelling older patients with type 2 dia-betes mellitus. Geriatr Gerontol Int 2017. [Epub ahead of print].
11. Lee SJ, Boscardin WJ, Stijacic Cenzer I, et al. The risks and benefits of imple-menting glycemic control guidelines in frail older adults with diabetes mellitus. J Am Geriatr Soc 2011;59(4):666–72.
12. Brown JS, Wing R, Barrett-Connor E, et al. Lifestyle intervention is associated with lower prevalence of urinary incontinence: the diabetes prevention program. Dia-betes Care 2006;29(2):385–90.
13. Diabetes Prevention Program Research Group, Knowler WC, Fowler SE, Hamman RF, et al. 10-year follow-up of diabetes incidence and weight loss in the Diabetes Prevention Program Outcomes Study. Lancet 2009;374(9702): 1677–86.
14. Florez H, Pan Q, Ackermann RT, et al. Impact of lifestyle intervention and metfor-min on health-related quality of life: the diabetes prevention program randomized trial. J Gen Intern Med 2012;27(12):1594–601.
15. Effect of intensive blood-glucose control with metformin on complications in over-weight patients with type 2 diabetes (UKPDS 34). UK Prospective Diabetes Study (UKPDS) Group. Lancet 1998;352(9131):854–65.
16. Intensive blood-glucose control with sulphonylureas or insulin compared with conventional treatment and risk of complications in patients with type 2 diabetes (UKPDS 33). UK Prospective Diabetes Study (UKPDS) Group. Lancet 1998; 352(9131):837–53.
17. Holman RR, Paul SK, Bethel MA, et al. 10-year follow-up of intensive glucose con-trol in type 2 diabetes. N Engl J Med 2008;359(15):1577–89.
18. Action to Control Cardiovascular Risk in Diabetes Study Group, Gerstein HC, Miller ME, Byington RP, et al. Effects of intensive glucose lowering in type 2 dia-betes. N Engl J Med 2008;358(24):2545–59.
19. Group AC, Patel A, MacMahon S, et al. Intensive blood glucose control and vascular outcomes in patients with type 2 diabetes. N Engl J Med 2008; 358(24):2560–72.
20. Duckworth W, Abraira C, Moritz T, et al. Glucose control and vascular complica-tions in veterans with type 2 diabetes. N Engl J Med 2009;360(2):129–39.
21. Duckworth WC, Abraira C, Moritz TE, et al. The duration of diabetes affects the response to intensive glucose control in type 2 subjects: the VA Diabetes Trial. J Diabetes Complications 2011;25(6):355–61.

22. Li Y, Burrows NR, Gregg EW, et al. Declining rates of hospitalization for nontraumatic lower-extremity amputation in the diabetic population aged 40 years or older: U.S., 1988-2008. Diabetes Care 2012;35(2):273–7.

23. US Centers for Disease Control and Prevention. Diabetes public health resource. Available at: https://www.cdc.gov/diabetes/statistics/hypoglycemia/fig5byage. htm. Accessed April 9, 2017.

24. Ferrannini E, Buzzigoli G, Bonadonna R, et al. Insulin resistance in essential hypertension. N Engl J Med 1987;317(6):350–7.

25. American Diabetes Association. (7) Approaches to glycemic treatment. Diabetes Care 2016;39(Suppl 1):S52–9.

26. Inzucchi SE, Bergenstal RM, Buse JB, et al. Management of hyperglycemia in type 2 diabetes: a patient-centered approach: position statement of the American Diabetes Association (ADA) and the European Association for the Study of Diabetes (EASD). Diabetes Care 2012;35(6):1364–79.

27. Umegaki H, Makino T, Uemura K, et al. The associations among insulin resistance, hyperglycemia, physical performance, diabetes mellitus, and cognitive function in relatively healthy older adults with subtle cognitive dysfunction. Front Aging Neurosci 2017;9:72.

28. Li W, Risacher SL, Huang E, et al. Alzheimer's disease neuroimaging I. Type 2 diabetes mellitus is associated with brain atrophy and hypometabolism in the ADNI cohort. Neurology 2016;87(6):595–600.

29. Borson S, Scanlan JM, Chen P, et al. The Mini-Cog as a screen for dementia: validation in a population-based sample. J Am Geriatr Soc 2003;51(10):1451–4.

30. Scanlan J, Borson S. The Mini-Cog: receiver operating characteristics with expert and naive raters. Int J Geriatr Psychiatry 2001;16(2):216–22.

31. Anderson RJ, Freedland KE, Clouse RE, et al. The prevalence of comorbid depression in adults with diabetes: a meta-analysis. Diabetes Care 2001;24(6): 1069–78.

32. Lustman PJ, Clouse RE. Treatment of depression in diabetes: impact on mood and medical outcome. J Psychosom Res 2002;53(4):917–24.

33. Badedi M, Solan Y, Darraj H, et al. Factors associated with long-term control of type 2 diabetes mellitus. J Diabetes Res 2016;2016:2109542.

34. Kirkman MS, Briscoe VJ, Clark N, et al. Diabetes in older adults: a consensus report. J Am Geriatr Soc 2012;60(12):2342–56.

35. Breuker C, Abraham O, di Trapanie L, et al. Patients with diabetes are at high risk of serious medication errors at hospital: interest of clinical pharmacist intervention to improve healthcare. Eur J Intern Med 2017;38:38–45.

36. Hong X, Chen X, Chu J, et al. Multiple diabetic complications, as well as impaired physical and mental function, are associated with declining balance function in older persons with diabetes mellitus. Clin Interv Aging 2017;12:189–95.

37. Schwartz AV, Vittinghoff E, Sellmeyer DE, et al. Diabetes-related complications, glycemic control, and falls in older adults. Diabetes Care 2008;31(3): 391–6.

38. Linde JM, Nijman RJ, Trzpis M, et al. Urinary incontinence in the Netherlands: prevalence and associated risk factors in adults. Neurourol Urodyn 2016. [Epub ahead of print].

39. Kane AE, Gregson E, Theou O, et al. The association between frailty, the metabolic syndrome, and mortality over the lifespan. Geroscience 2017;39(2): 221–9.

40. Perez-Tasigchana RF, Leon-Munoz LM, Lopez-Garcia E, et al. Metabolic syndrome and insulin resistance are associated with frailty in older adults: a prospective cohort study. Age Ageing 2017;1–6.
41. McAlister FA, Youngson E, Eurich DT. Treated glycosylated hemoglobin levels in individuals with diabetes mellitus vary little by health status: a retrospective cohort study. Medicine (Baltimore) 2016;95(24):e3894.

40.

41.

Hormone Replacement
The Fountain of Youth?

Bradley R. Williams, PharmD, BCGP[a],*, Janet Soojeung Cho, PharmD, CDE, BCGP[b]

KEYWORDS

- Older adults • Hormone replacement therapy • Antiaging • Menopause
- Andropause • Sexual function

KEY POINTS

- Hormones and hormone precursors have been investigated as antiaging treatments to delay the onset or progression of age-associated changes in body composition, strength, and physical and cognitive function.
- Dehydroepiandrosterone and growth hormone have been investigated. Most studies have included small sample sizes and have been of short duration. Results have generally been mixed, at best.
- Menopausal hormone therapy (MHT) is effective in treating vasomotor and genitourinary symptoms of menopause in women. However, due to safety considerations, patients require individualized treatment and need to evaluate the risks and benefits before MHT use.
- Testosterone has been shown to be effective in older men with hypogonadism who have demonstrated declines in physiologic function. Clinical practice guidelines for appropriate diagnosis and treatment have been published.
- The lack of clinical studies evaluating the long-term effects and risks of hormone replacement for antiaging indications limit its use.

INTRODUCTION

One need only to look at advertising in mass media to recognize that aging is frequently viewed as a health condition that can be remedied by any number of products, from pills to injections to creams and lotions. It often seems that a major goal in life is to age while remaining young (Dorian Gray, anyone?). Toward that end, medical science has brought us hormones, hormone precursors, hormone analogs, and several other products to help people achieve that goal. For some, aging and

The authors have no relevant conflicts to disclose.
[a] Titus Family Department of Clinical Pharmacy, University of Southern California, School of Pharmacy, 1985 Zonal Avenue, Los Angeles, CA 90089-9121, USA; [b] USC Specialty Pharmacy, University of Southern California, School of Pharmacy, 1000 South Fremont Avenue, A-10, Suite 10150, Alhambra, CA 91803, USA
* Corresponding author.
E-mail address: bradwill@usc.edu

appearance are equated with health status.[1] Antiaging is viewed by many as success-ful aging.[2] Supplements and other products are heavily advertised, promising to restore youthful function. These include growth hormone (https://www.youtube. com/watch?v=CGevQwAYnJo), dehydroepiandrosterone (DHEA) (https://www. youtube.com/watch?v=fqBMXqg8XYM), testosterone supplements (https://www. youtube.com/watch?v=SBx1Cn_GmK4), and female hormone replacement products (https://www.youtube.com/watch?v=OBW-C31uTyM).

Natural aging is accompanied by reduced production of growth hormone and sex hormones. The reductions begin in middle age, with noticeable physiologic changes becoming evident by the sixth or seventh decade of life. The changes are responsible for lost muscle mass, reduced energy, exercise capacity, and alterations in sexual function. Several factors are responsible for these changes.

Although some form of hormone replacement therapy (HRT) for women has been prescribed for nearly a century, the use of DHEA, growth hormone, and testosterone for men, has been much more recent.[3] There remains much controversy regarding the benefits and risks associated with these treatments. This article reviews the available evidence of therapeutic efficacy and the adverse effects of the more commonly used agents.

Dehydroepiandrosterone

DHEA, a precursor of steroidogenesis, is secreted by the adrenal glands. It is metab-olized to androstenedione, which in turn is metabolized to estrone and estradiol in women, and to testosterone in men. DHEA production peaks in early adulthood and declines over time.

The use of DHEA to affect the physical aging process was sparked by results of an-imal studies, which demonstrated prevention of cancer, heart disease, diabetes, and obesity, as well as positive effects on the immune system. It also has been shown in animal models to improve survival of central neurons and glial cells, and improve learning and memory.[4] Because it is metabolized to testosterone and estradiol, DHEA has also generated interest as a potential therapy to reverse age-associated declines in sex hormones.

Several studies have been conducted in humans to evaluate the effect of DHEA on several aspects of physical and cognitive aging. Results have been mixed, at best, with few studies identifying any major positive effect (**Table 1**). Most studies have included small samples and have been of short duration. In addition, several other methodological reasons have been identified as constraints to obtaining consistent re-sults in humans, including differences between animal and human models, doses used in studies, effects of aging and comorbidities, and variability in what is consid-ered a normal DHEA serum value.[5] In general, although relatively free of significant adverse effects in doses of 100 mg/d or less, DHEA has not been found to produce notable benefit to reverse the effect of aging.[4,6,7] Additionally, the Beers Criteria for Potentially Inappropriate Medications (PIMs) Use in Older Adults recommends avoid-ing the use of growth hormone, except as hormone replacement after pituitary gland removal.[8]

Growth Hormone

Growth hormone and insulin-like growth factor-1 decline with advancing age, leading to metabolic disorders, including insulin resistance, cardiovascular changes, and increased frailty.[21] The decline in growth hormone secretion is accompanied by an alteration in release pattern, resulting in altered effects. From peak levels, growth hor-mone secretion may decline by as much as 70% by the eighth decade of life.[21]

Table 1
Dehydroepiandrosterone effects

Reference	Participants	Design	Intervention	Outcome
Morales et al,[9] 1994	13 M; 17 W 40–70 y	R, DB, PC, CO	50 mg/d × 6 mo	Improved physical and psychological well-being
Wolf et al,[10] 1997	25 M; 15 W M: 69.4 ± 1.2 y W: 69.1 ± 1.7 y	R, DB, PC, CO	50 mg/d × 2 wk	No change in mood or cognition
Labrie et al,[11] 1997	W: 14 60–70 y	OL, RM	10% w/v cream q day × 12 mo	Improvement in vaginal epithelium No effect on endometrial epithelium Increased BMD
Flynn et al,[12] 1999	M: 39 60–84 y	R, DB, PC, CO	100 mg/d × 3 mo	No change in well-being No change in body composition
Reiter et al,[13] 1999	M: 40 (30 completed) 41–69 y	R, DB, PC	50 mg/d × 6 mo	Improved scores on IIEF questionnaire
Baulieu et al,[14] 2000	M: 140 W: 140 60–79 y	R, DB, PC, PG	50 mg/d × 12 mo	Improved well-being Increased sex hormones, no change in libido or sexual function Reduced bone turnover in women >70 y
Arlt et al,[15] 2001	M: 22 50–69 y	R, DB, PC, CO	50 mg/d × 4 mo	No change in mood No effect on sexuality No effect on serum lipids, bone markers, body composition, exercise capacity
van Niekerk et al,[16] 2001	M: 41 ≥60 y	R, DB, PC, CO	50 mg/d × 13 wk	No change in mood or cognition
Villareal & Holloszy,[17] 2004	M: 28 W: 28 65–78 y	R, DB, PC	50 mg/d × 6 mo	Reduced SC fat Increased insulin sensitivity
Nair et al,[6] 2006	M: 87 W: 57 ≥60 y	R, DB, PC	75 mg/d × 2 y (M) 50 mg/d × 2 y (W)	No change in QoL Increased BMD
Igwebuike et al,[18] 2008	W: 31 54–72 y	R, DB, PC	50 mg/d × 12 wk	No improvement in physical performance or insulin sensitivity No change in body composition

(continued on next page)

Table 1 (continued)				
Reference	Participants	Design	Intervention	Outcome
Weiss et al,[19] 2009	M: 55 W: 58 65–75 y	R, PC (year 1) OL (year 2)	50 mg/d	M: No change in BMD or bone turnover W: Increased spine BMD and reduced bone turnover
Merritt et al,[20] 2012	W: 48 55–80 y	DB, PC, CO	50 mg/d × 4 wk	No effect on cognitive tests

Abbreviations: BMD, bone mineral density; CO, cross-over; DB, double-blind; IIEF, International Index of Erectile Function; M, men; OL, open-label; PC, placebo-controlled; q day, daily; QoL, quality of life; R, randomized; RM, repeated measures; SC, subcutaneous; W, women; W/V, weight/volume.
   Data from Refs.[6,9–20]

Age-associated changes, including an increase and redistribution of body fat, reduced bone density, and reduced muscle mass and strength has spurred interest in growth hormone treatment in older adults.[22] These changes mimic what is observed in younger individuals with growth hormone deficiency. Endocrine Society guidelines for the use of growth hormone in adults are limited to its use in adults with growth hormone deficiency, and make no recommendation for use in others.[23] Whether use of growth hormone in healthy older adults will produce results similar to those seen in growth hormone-deficient individuals is controversial.[22,24]

Clinical studies have evaluated the effect of growth hormone on several aspects of age-associated changes, including effects on lean body mass, body fat, bone density, muscle strength and function (Table 2). Although numerous studies have demonstrated improvement in some areas, increased physical function has not generally been found.[24–26]

Adverse effects of growth hormone identified in trials include malaise, joint stiffness, arthralgias, glucose intolerance, and lower extremity edema.[24,27,28] Use is contraindicated in those with active malignancies. Use in people with diabetes may require adjustment of antidiabetes medications. Thyroid and adrenal function should be routinely monitored during growth hormone therapy.[23]

Hormone Replacement in Women

HRT has been used for several decades for the treatment of climacteric syndrome in women. Estrogen preparations were first commercially available in 1926 and evolved as a regular part of medical practice in some developed countries by the 1970s.[3] Some believed that all aspects of aging were in some way related to the decline of estrogens in the body and by administration of estrogens, the effects of aging may be slowed.[32] Later, based on epidemiologic data in the 1990s demonstrating a protective effect of estrogen on the heart and bone,[33–35] it was common for HRT to be prescribed for prevention of coronary heart disease and osteoporosis.

Beginning in the late 1990s, multiple clinical studies revealed new findings and risks of HRT, leading to a shift toward conservative HRT use. The Heart and Estrogen/progestin Replacement Study (HERS) on HRT found no reduction of the risk for coronary heart disease as secondary prevention in postmenopausal women. Rather, there was an increased rate of thromboembolic events and gall bladder disease.[36–38] The Women's Health Initiative (WHI) conducted 2 studies to evaluate the use of combined estrogen and progestin, and estrogen alone, in postmenopausal women. Both studies

Table 2
Growth hormone effects

Reference	Participants	Design	Intervention	Outcome
Papadakis et al,[27] 1996	M: 52 70–85 y Low IGF-1 levels	R, DB, PC	0.03 mg/kg TIW × 6 mo	Increased LBM Decreased fat mass No change in strength or endurance No change in cognitive function
Blackman et al,[29] 2002	M: 74 W: 57 65–88 y	R, DB, PC, PG	GH: 30 mcg/kg TIW ± sex hormone × 26 wk	Increased IGF-1 Increased LBM Decreased fat mass
Franco et al,[28] 2005	W: 40 (35 completed) 51–63 y	R, DB, PC	0.67 mg SC × 12 mo	Reduced visceral fat Improved lipid profile Increased insulin sensitivity
Giannoulis et al,[30] 2006	M: 80 65–80 y	R, DB, PC	GH up to 1.2 mg/d ± Testosterone × 6 mo	Increased IGF-1 Increased LBM
Sathiavageeswaran et al,[31] 2007	M: 22 W: 12 60–77 y	R, DB, PC	GH, targeted to normal-for-age IGF-1 levels	Increased IGF-1 No change in mood or cognitive function

Abbreviations: IGF-1, insulin-like growth factor-1; LBM, lean body mass; PG, parallel group; TIW, 3 times weekly.
Data from Refs.[27–31]

ended prematurely due to excess risk of thromboembolic disease. The estrogen plus progestin study found increased risk for breast cancer as well.[39,40] The WHI trials demonstrated that the health risks exceeded benefits from use of HRT in the forms of estrogen plus progestin and estrogen alone.

Since the published findings of the HERS studies and WHI trials, the use of HRT in women aged 40 year or older dropped significantly in the United States. According to the National Health and Nutrition Examination Survey, oral HRT use decreased from 22% in 1999 to 2002 down to 4.7% by 2009 to 2010.[41] Additionally, HRT use in older women was no longer recommended for preventative measures but mainly for the management and symptomatic relief of severe menopausal symptoms.

HRT remains a controversial topic yet continues to be a cornerstone of antiaging practices and the media to help reverse effects of aging and to improve quality of life.[25] The decrease in hormone production with age has been related to decrease in intellectual activity, mood, lean body mass, bone mineral density, and skin aging.[42,43] Off-label uses of hormones have been observed for possible benefits in mood, dementia, bone health, diabetes, colorectal cancer, endometrial cancer, and antiaging in skin.

CURRENT HORMONE REPLACEMENT THERAPY GUIDELINES AND RESEARCH (WOMEN)

The use of hormone replacement in women is primarily indicated for the management of severe menopausal symptoms, specifically vasomotor and genitourinary, and is now referred to as menopausal hormone therapy (MHT). Clinical guidelines for MHT have been published by the Endocrine Society.[44]

Vasomotor Symptoms

Vasomotor symptoms (VMS) include the classic menopause symptoms of hot flashes (also referenced as hot flushes), cold sweats, and night sweats,[45] and are prevalent during and following menopause. In the United States, nearly 75% of postmenopausal women experience VMS[46] and symptoms last more than 1 year, typically 2 to 4 years, for most women.[47] For symptomatic menopausal women, estrogen therapy is considered the most effective treatment to reduce VMS and improve quality of life.[48,49]

Genitourinary Syndrome of Menopause

Genitourinary syndrome of menopause (GSM) is the term that encompasses vulvovaginal atrophy (eg, vulvar pain, burning, itching, vaginal dryness, vaginal discharge, dyspareunia, and spotting or bleeding after intercourse) and urinary tract dysfunction (eg, dysuria, recurrent urinary tract infections, and urinary frequency). Both local vaginal estrogen therapy and systemic MHT therapy may be used for GSM.[50,51]

RISKS OF MENOPAUSAL HORMONE THERAPY

MHT is beneficial in the treatment of VMS and GSM; however it poses serious health risks. Various studies report increased risks of breast cancer, stroke, venous thromboembolic events, gallbladder disease, and incontinence with the use of estrogen plus progestin.[52,53] Additionally, increased risk for endometrial hyperplasia and cancer is seen with unopposed estrogen therapy in women with an intact uterus, as well as reported probable increased risk of developing dementia as seen in the WHI Memory Study (WHIMS). These findings led to multiple US boxed warnings on estrogens and progestins.[44,48] An individual risk assessment, along with a comparison with appropriate population-related data and studies, is essential to make the best clinical decision in MHT use.

RISK CALCULATIONS

Newly added to the 2015 Endocrine Society Clinical Practice Guideline for MHT, calculations for cardiovascular risk and breast cancer risk may be referenced before considering MHT.[44,54] These tools may aid the clinician and patient in discussing risks and benefits, and facilitate shared decision-making.

When considering cardiovascular risk, the clinical practice guideline is based on the American College of Cardiology and American Heart Association cardiovascular disease (CVD) risk calculations[55]:

- Low 10-year CVD risk (<10%): MHT okay
- Moderate 10-year CVD risk (5%–10%): MHT okay, consider transdermal formulation
- High 10-year CVD risk (>10%): avoid MHT.

Breast Cancer Risk

Recommend the following, based on 5-year National Cancer Institute or International Breast Intervention Study (IBIS) Breast Cancer Risk Assessment[44]:

- Low breast cancer risk (<1.67%): MHT okay
- Intermediate breast cancer risk (1.67%–5%): caution for MHT
- High breast cancer risk (>5%): avoid MHT.

RECOMMENDATIONS FOR MENOPAUSAL HORMONE THERAPY

The recommendation for use of MHT for VMS and GSM relief are for healthy women, without contraindications (**Box 1**) or excess cardiovascular or breast cancer risks, and age less than 60 years or less than 10 years after menopause onset.[44] In this specific age range population, the benefits of MHT seem to outweigh the risks. The guidelines recommend choosing and tailoring MHT to the individual patient based on severity of symptoms, patient-specific factors, and risk and benefit of therapy. The Beers Criteria PIMs recommends avoiding oral or transdermal patch estrogens with or without progestins (vaginal creams or tablets are considered acceptable for lower urinary track symptoms).[8] The decision to use PIMs in older adults is highly individual, taking into consideration comorbidity burden, frailty, and risk of adverse effects.

When selecting the MHT dose, type, route of administration, and duration of therapy, the following main concepts may help in navigating clinical decision-making:

- Use the lowest effective dose
- Women with intact uterus should be given estrogen plus progestin combination therapy
- Women without intact uterus may be given unopposed estrogen therapy
- Patients with higher risk factors may alternatively use nonoral-route MHT
- Use the shortest duration of therapy, with a maximum duration of 5 years.

Box 1
Menopausal hormone therapy contraindications

Absolute contraindications

- Undiagnosed abnormal genital bleeding
- Active or history of deep vein thrombosis or pulmonary embolism
- Active or recent arterial thromboembolic disease (ie, stroke, myocardial infarction)
- Known thrombophilic disorders
- Known liver dysfunction or disease
- Known, suspected, or history of breast cancer
- Known or suspected estrogen-dependent or progesterone-dependent neoplasia
- Known or suspected pregnancy

Relative contraindications

- Hypertriglyceridemia
- Gall bladder disease
- Hypoparathyroidism (risk for severe hypocalcemia)
- High risk of heart disease (including elevated blood pressure, history of fluid retention)
- Intermediate or high risk of breast cancer
- Benign meningioma
- May exacerbate asthma, diabetes mellitus, migraine, systemic lupus erythematosus, epilepsy, porphyria, or hepatic hemangioma.

Data from Stuenkel CA, Davis SR, Gompel A, et al. Treatment of symptoms of the menopause: an Endocrine Society clinical practice guideline. J Clin Endocrinol Metab 2015;100:3975–4011; and Santen RJ, Allred DC, Ardoin SP, et al. Postmenopausal hormone therapy: an Endocrine Society scientific statement. J Clin Endocrinol Metab 2010;95:s1–66.

OFF-LABEL USE OF MENOPAUSAL HORMONE THERAPY

Several studies allude to other potential benefits and preventative benefits of MHT.

Potential Benefits of Menopausal Hormone Therapy

Other potential benefits of MHT that have been investigated include conditions related to menopause, such as sleep disruption, anxiety and depressive symptoms, and arthralgia. **Table 3** describes related studies and their findings.

Potential Preventative Benefits of Menopausal Hormone Therapy

The most recent MHT clinical practice guideline from the Endocrine Society does not recommend the use of MHT for chronic disease prevention, such as CVD, osteoporosis, and dementia. This is in line with the findings from the WHI postintervention follow-up of the WHI hormone therapy studies.[53] However, various studies show other potential preventative benefits of MHT. **Table 4** shows a list of studies related to positive results for MHT and colorectal cancer, endometrial cancer, bone fractures, and type 2 diabetes.[48]

Uncertain Benefits

Although there is less evidence that MHT is beneficial for reversing skin aging and improving cognition, some may still use hormone therapy for various antiaging uses. **Table 5** includes studies that evaluated the potential benefits of MHT in regard to antiaging targets.

Table 3
Potential benefits of menopausal hormone therapy (sleep, anxiety and depression, arthralgia)

Reference	Participants	Design	Intervention	Outcomes
Barnabei et al,[49] 2005 WHI	W: 16,608 Postmenopausal with intact uterus 50–79 y	R, DB, PC	0.625 mg CEE + 2.5 mg MPA daily × mean follow-up time 5.6 y	Relief of joint pain or stiffness and general aches or pains
Manson et al,[53] 2013 WHI	W: 27,347 Postmenopausal with intact uterus 50–79 y	R, DB, PC	0.625 mg CEE + 2.5 mg MPA daily × mean follow-up time 5.6 y OR 0.625 mg CEE daily × mean follow-up time 5.6 y	Significantly fewer sleep disturbances
Gleason et al,[56] 2015	W: 693 Postmenopausal with intact uterus Mean age: 52.6 y	R, DB, PC	0.45 mg CEE + 200 mg micronized progesterone every first 12 d of each month × 4 y OR 50 mcg transdermal estradiol + 200 mg micronized progesterone every first 12 d of each month × 4 y	Small improvements in depression and anxiety symptoms

Abbreviations: CEE, conjugated equine estrogen; MPA, medroxyprogesterone acetate.
Data from Refs.[49,53,56]

Table 4
Potential preventative benefits of menopausal hormone therapy (colorectal cancer, endometrial cancer, bone health and fractures, type 2 diabetes)

Reference	Participants	Design	Intervention	Outcomes
Chlebowski et al,[57] 2004 WHI	W: 16,608 Postmenopausal with intact uterus 50–79 y	R, DB, PC	0.625 mg CEE + 2.5 mg MPA daily × mean follow-up time 5.6 y	Short-term hormone use associated with a decreased risk of colorectal cancer Colorectal cancers in treatment arm were diagnosed at a more advanced stage compared with placebo
Anderson et al,[58] 2003 WHI	W: 16,608 Postmenopausal with intact uterus 50–79 y	R, DB, PC	0.625 mg CEE + 2.5 mg MPA daily × mean follow-up time 5.6 y	Similar rates of endometrial cancer
Cauley et al,[59] 2003 WHI	W: 16,608 Postmenopausal with intact uterus 50–79 y	R, DB, PC	0.625 mg CEE + 2.5 mg MPA daily × mean follow-up time 5.6 y	Increased total hip BMD Reduced risk of factures
Kanaya et al,[60] 2003	W: 2763 Postmenopausal established CHD <80 y	R, DB, PC	0.625 mg CEE + 2.5 mg MPA daily × 4.1 y	Reduced the incidence of diabetes by 35%
Margolis et al,[61] 2004 WHI	W: 15,641 Postmenopausal with intact uterus 50–79 y	R, DB, PC	0.625 mg CEE + 2.5 mg MPA daily × mean follow-up time 5.6 y	In the first year follow-up, a significant fall in insulin resistance was seen

Abbreviation: CHD, coronary heart disease.
Data from Refs.[57–61]

Hormone Replacement in Men

In addition to treatment of hypogonadism in men, hormone replacement has been promoted for improving function or maintaining quality of life by avoiding the symptoms associated with aging, such as decreased strength, energy, and libido.[2] For many years, testosterone was available only by injection, including long-acting depot formulations. Dosing by this route resulted in high peak hormone levels that could lead to severe adverse effects, including testicular atrophy and hepatic damage. With the advent of topical agents, prescribing of testosterone products to older men has significantly increased.[66] The change may be, at least in part, because lower and more sustained levels were possible, reducing the risk for many adverse events.

Testosterone, like other hormones, is secreted in a circadian pattern with peak levels occurring in the morning. After early adulthood, secretion declines but still remains in the normal range for most men at least until old age. The decline is accompanied by a rise in sex hormone binding globulin, which reduces the available amount of free testosterone.[67] When total testosterone levels are considered, levels consistent

Table 5
Effects of menopausal hormone therapy on skin and cognition

Reference	Participants	Design	Intervention	Outcomes
Phillips et al,[62] 2008	W: 485 Postmenopausal with intact uterus, with aging skin 45–67 y	R, DB, DD, PC	1 mg NA + 5 mcg EE daily OR 1 mg NA + 10 mcg EE daily × 48 wk	No significant effect in mild to moderate age-related facial skin changes
Rittié et al,[63] 2008	W: 40 Postmenopausal Mean age 75 y M: 30 Mean age 75 y With photodamaged skin	CS	Topical estradiol strengths of 0.01%, 0.1%, 1%, 2.5% applied to aged (hip) or photoaged skin (facial or forearm) × 2 wk	Topical estrogen treatment stimulated collagen production in sun-protected hip skin. No effect on facial or forearm skin.
Maki et al,[64] 2007	W: 180 Postmenopausal 45–55 y Note: Study terminated early due to findings from WHI	R, DB, PC	0.625 mg CEE + 2.5 mg MPA daily × 4 mo	No differences on any cognitive or QoL measures Potential negative effects on verbal memory
Espeland et al,[65] 2004 WHIMS	W: 2947 Postmenopausal With prior hysterectomy 65–79 y	R, DB, PC	0.625 mg CEE daily	Lower global cognitive function scores

Abbreviations: CS, cohort study; DD, double dummy; EE, ethinyl estradiol; NA, norethindrone acetate; WHIMS, Woman's Health Initiative Memory Study.
Data from Refs.[62–65]

with hypogonadism are found in nearly one-third of men by age 70 years and approximately one-half by age 80 years.[68] Symptomatic hypogonadism, however, is much less prevalent, occurring in less than 20% of 70 year-old men.[69] Proposed criteria for the diagnosis of late-onset hypogonadism include reduced total (<11 nmol/L) and free (<220 pmol/L) testosterone in the presence of at least 3 sexual symptoms.[70] Other signs and symptoms, including reduced energy and exercise tolerance, depressed mood, and cognitive changes, are encountered as part of normal aging and are thus too nonspecific to be of diagnostic value.[67]

The Endocrine Society published updated guidelines for the treatment of androgen deficiency in men. Diagnosis should be pursued in men with multiple symptoms of deficiency. Laboratory evaluation should include repeated morning total and free testosterone levels, along with follicle-stimulating hormone and luteinizing hormone levels to differentiate other potential causes, and bone density in those with a fracture history. Goals of therapy include improved sexual function, increased bone density, and increased sense of well-being. Treatment should not be initiated in men with active prostate or breast cancer, and caution should be used in those with an elevated prostate specific antigen or a strong family history of prostate cancer. The guideline specifically recommends against initiation of testosterone therapy in older men solely in the presence of reduced testosterone levels.[71]

Table 6
Testosterone replacement therapy

Reference	Participants	Design	Intervention	Outcome
Mårin et al,[77] 1993	M: 31 ≥40 y (Mean: 57.7 ± 2.1) Abdominal obesity BMI <35 Low serum testosterone	R, DB, PC, PG	Gel, 125 mg/d (1 testosterone product and 1 dihydrotestosterone product) × 9 mo	Decreased visceral fat in testosterone group
Snyder et al,[78] 1999	M: 108 ≥65 y Low or normal testosterone at baseline	R, DB, PC	Patch, 6 mg/d × 36 mo	Increased BMD in only in those with low testosterone at baseline
English et al,[79] 2000	M: 46 Mean 62 ± 2 y Chronic stable angina	R, DB, PC	Patch, 5 mg/d × 2 wk	Increased time to ST-segment depression No change in angina frequency
Kenny et al,[80] 2001	M: 67 44 completers 65–87 y Low serum testosterone	R, DB, PC	Patch, 5 mg/d × 12 mo	Increased LBM Reduced body fat Maintained bone density
Aversa et al,[81] 2003	M: 20 48–66 y Arteriogenic ED with sildenafil nonresponse	R, PC	Patch, 5 mg/d × 30 d Sildenafil to both groups	Improved penile blood flow Reduced ED symptoms
Steidle et al,[82] 2003	M: 406 20–80 y (Mean 58.0 ± 10.3)	R, DB, PC, AC OL for patch	Gel: 50 or 100 mg/d × 90 d Patch: 5 mg/d × 90 d	Increased LBM and decreased body fat vs placebo and patch for 100 mg gel dose Improved erection, desire, motivation, performance vs placebo for 100 mg gel dose
Shabsigh et al,[83] 2004	M: 75 26–79 y (Mean 59.7 ± 9.8) Hypogonadal ED unresponsive to sildenafil	R, DB, PC, PG	Gel, 5 gm/day × 12 wk Sildenafil to both groups	Improved erectile function at week 4, but not at weeks 8 or 12 No significant change in IIEF scores

(continued on next page)

Table 6
(continued)

Reference	Participants	Design	Intervention	Outcome
Seftel et al,[84] 2004	M: 406 20–80 y (Mean 58.0 ± 10.3)	R, DB, PC, AC OL for patch	Gel: 50 or 100 mg/d × 90 d Patch: 5 mg/d × 90 d	Increased erections and intercourse frequency at 30 and 90 d vs placebo for 100 mg dose Increased desire and nighttime erections at 90 d vs placebo for 100 mg dose
Srinivas-Shankar et al,[85] 2010	M: 274 ≥65 y Frail, low or low-normal total serum testosterone	R, DB, PC, PG	Gel, 50 mg/d × 6 mo	Increased LBM Reduced fat mass Improvement on Aging Males Symptom scale
Cunningham et al,[86] 2016 (TT)	M: 470 ≥65 y Low testosterone with and low libido	R, DB, PC, PG	Gel 1%, adjusted to achieve normal testosterone levels × 12 mo	Improved sexual desire and activity No effect on erectile function No threshold testosterone level observed for any outcome
Roy et al,[87] 2017 (TT)	M: 126 ≥65 y Low testosterone with unexplained anemia	R, DB, PC, PG	Gel 1%, adjusted to achieve normal testosterone levels × 12 mo	Improved hemoglobin Resolved anemia
Resnick et al,[88] 2017 (TT)	M: 493 ≥65 y Low testosterone with age-associated memory impairment	R, DB, PC, PG	Gel 1%, adjusted to achieve normal testosterone levels × 12 mo	No change in paragraph recall No change in visual memory, executive function or spatial ability
Budoff et al,[89] 2017 (xx)	M: 138 ≥65 y Low testosterone with sexual dysfunction, physical dysfunction, and/or reduced vitality	R, DB, PC, PG	Gel 1%, adjusted to achieve normal testosterone levels × 12 mo	Increased noncalcified arterial plaque and total plaque volumes
Snyder et al,[90] 2017 (xx)	M: 211 ≥65 y Low testosterone with T-score ≥-3.0	R, DB, PC, PG	Gel 1%, adjusted to achieve normal testosterone levels × 12 mo	Increased volumetric BMD Increased bone strength (trabecular>peripheral; spine>hip

Abbreviations: AC, active control; BMI, body mass index; ED, erectile dysfunction; OL, open label; TT, testosterone trial.
Data from Refs.[77–90]

Dating back to the 1980s, many clinical trials have investigated the use of testosterone; the older trials were conducted before the availability of transdermal formulations.[72] These formulations have replaced injectable, implantable, and oral dosage forms in an overwhelming number of cases.[66] **Table 6** includes clinical trials conducted using the current standard dosage forms. In an effort to systematically evaluate testosterone treatment, a series of 7 coordinated trials (Testosterone Trials) have been initiated.[73] Results from some of the trials are noted in **Table 6**.

Although study protocols and sample sizes vary considerably, there are consistent findings of increased lean body mass, decreased fat, and maintained or increased bone density in older men with low serum testosterone levels but not in those with normal levels. There is no consistency regarding increased muscle strength or physical or cognitive function. Results with the newer topical agents are similar to those reported in studies using intramuscular or oral preparations.[74]

Commonly encountered adverse effects include increased hematocrit and prostate specific antigen levels. It is recommended that both be routinely monitored in men taking testosterone supplements.[74,75] An increased risk for adverse cardiovascular events has been reported but has not been a consistent finding.[76]

SUMMARY

As long as people continue to resist the normal aging process, there will be interest in maintaining a younger appearance and function. Although older adults with true hormone deficiencies that adversely affect their function to the degree that their daily activities and interests are compromised may be appropriate candidates for treatment, those with normal functional capacities are not. There is little evidence of benefit for treatment with DHEA or growth hormone beyond those with documented deficiencies.

MHT has clear and effective benefits in treating vasomotor and genitourinary symptoms of menopause in women but also carries multiple safety concerns, which require a risk versus benefit evaluation. Women with severe symptoms should be offered a trial of low-dose hormone therapy, with re-evaluation on a periodic basis to monitor for adverse outcomes.

Men with symptomatic hypogonadism likewise should be offered a trial of testosterone. Improvement in symptoms and metabolic indices that restore normal function are appropriate outcomes. Routine assessment for increased hematocrit and prostate cancer are appropriate monitoring procedures.

The use of hormone therapy in antiaging indications, however, is limited due to the lack of strong clinical studies evaluating the efficacy, risks, and long-term effects. Until clear benefit is demonstrated, routine prescribing for these indications is not warranted.

REFERENCES

1. Calasanti T, King N, Pietilä I, et al. Rationales for anti-aging activities in middle age: aging, health, or appearance? Gerontologist 2016;1–9. http://dx.doi.org/10.1093/geront/gnw111.
2. Flatt MA, Settersten RA, Ponsaran R, et al. Are "anti-aging medicine" and "successful aging" two sides of the same coin? Views of anti-aging practitioners. J Gerontol B Psychol Sci Soc Sci 2013;68:944–55.
3. VanKeep PA. The history and rationale of hormone replacement therapy. Maturitas 1990;12:163–70.
4. Legrain S, Girard L. Pharmacology and therapeutic effects of dehydroepiandrosterone in older subjects. Drugs Aging 2003;20:949–67.

5. Rutkowski K, Sowa P, Rutkowska-Talipsa J, et al. Dehydroepiandrosterone (DHEA): hypes and hopes. Drugs 2014;74:1195–207.

6. Nair KS, Rizza RA, O'Brien P, et al. DHEA in elderly women and DHEA or testosterone in elderly men. N Engl J Med 2006;355:1647–59.

7. Davis SR, Panjari M, Stanczyk FC. DHEA replacement for postmenopausal women. J Clin Endocrinol Metab 2011;96:1642–53.

8. American Geriatrics Society Expert Panel. American Geriatrics Society 2015 updated beers criteria for potentially inappropriate medication use in older adults. J Am Geriatr Soc 2015;63:2227–46.

9. Morales AJ, Nolan JJ, Nelson JC, et al. Effects of replacement dose of dehydroepiandrosterone in men and women of advancing age. J Clin Endocrinol Metab 1994;78:1360–7.

10. Wolf OT, Neumann O, Hellhamer DH, et al. Effects of a two-week physiological dehydroepiandrosterone substitution on cognitive performance and well-being in healthy elderly women and men. J Clin Endocrinol Metab 1997;82:2363–7.

11. Labrie F, Diamond P, Cusan L, et al. Effect of 12-month dehydroepiandrosterone replacement therapy on bone, vagina, and endometrium in postmenopausal women. J Clin Endocrinol Metab 1997;82:3498–505.

12. Flynn MA, Weaver-Osterholz D, Sharpe-Timms KL, et al. Dehydroepiandrosterone replacement in aging humans. J Clin Endocrinol Metab 1999;84:1527–33.

13. Reiter WJ, Pycha A, Schatzl G, et al. Dehydroepiandrosterone in the treatment of erectile dysfunction: a prospective, double-blind, randomized, placebo-controlled study. Urology 1999;53:590–5.

14. Baulieu EE, Thomas G, Legrain S, et al. Dehydroepiandrosterone (DHEA), DHEA sulfate, and aging: contribution of the DHEAge study to a sociobiomedical issue. Proc Natl Acad Sci U S A 2000;97:4279–84.

15. Arlt W, Callies F, Koehler I, et al. Dehydroepiandrosterone supplementation in healthy men with an age-related decline of dehydroepiandrosterone secretion. J Clin Endocrinol Metab 2001;86:4686–92.

16. van Niekerk JK, Huppert FA, Herbert J. Salivary cortisol and DHEA: association with measures of cognition and well-being in normal older men, and effects of three months of DHEA supplementation. Psychoneuroendocrinology 2001;26:591–612.

17. Villareal DT, Holloszy JO. Effect of DHEA on abdominal fat and insulin action in elderly women and men: a randomized controlled trial. JAMA 2004;292:2243–8.

18. Igwebuike A, Irving BA, Bigelow ML, et al. Lack of dehydroepiandrosterone effect on a combined endurance and exercise resistance program in postmenopausal women. J Clin Endocrinol Metab 2008;93:534–8.

19. Weiss EP, Shah K, Fontana L, et al. Dehydroepiandrosterone replacement therapy in older adults: 1- and 2-y effects on bone. Am J Clin Nutr 2009;89:1459–67.

20. Merritt P, Stangl B, Hirshman E, et al. Administration of dehydroepiandrosterone (DHEA) increases serum levels of androgens and estrogens but does not enhance short-term memory in post-menopausal women. Brain Res 2012;1483:54–62.

21. Giannoulis MF, Martin FC, Nair KS, et al. Hormone replacement therapy and physical function in healthy older men. Time to talk hormones? Endocr Rev 2012;33:314–77.

22. Nass R. Growth hormone access and aging. Endocrinol Metab Clin N Am 2013;42:187–99.

23. Molitch ME, Clemmons DR, Malozowski S, et al. Evaluation and treatment of adult growth hormone deficiency: an Endocrine Society clinical practice guideline. J Clin Endocrinol Metab 2011;96:1587–609.

24. Liu H, Bravada DM, Olkin I, et al. Systematic review: the safety and efficacy of growth hormone in the healthy elderly. Ann Intern Med 2007;146:104–15.

25. Samaras N, Papadopoulou MA, Samaras D, et al. Off-label use of hormones as an antiaging strategy: a review. Clin Interv Aging 2014;9:1175–86.

26. Sattler FR. Growth hormone in the aging male. Best Pract Res Clin Endocrinol Metab 2013;27:541–55.

27. Papadakis MA, Grady D, Black D, et al. Growth hormone replacement in healthy older men improves body composition but not functional ability. Ann Intern Med 1996;124:708–16.

28. Franco C, Brandberg J, Lönn L, et al. Growth hormone treatment reduces abdominal visceral fat in postmenopausal women with abdominal obesity: a 12-month placebo-controlled trial. J Clin Endocrinol Metab 2005;90:1466–74.

29. Blackman GH, Sorkin JD, Münzer T, et al. Growth hormone and sex steroid administration in healthy aged women and men. JAMA 2002;288:2282–92.

30. Giannoulis MG, Sonksen PH, Umpleby M, et al. The effects of growth hormone and/or testosterone in healthy elderly men: a randomized controlled trial. J Clin Endocrinol Metab 2006;91:477–84.

31. Sathiavageeswaran M, Burman P, Lawrence D, et al. Effects of GH on cognitive function in elderly patients with adult-onset GH deficiency: a placebo-controlled 12-month study. Eur J Endocrinol 2007;156:439–47.

32. Wilson RA. Feminine forever. London: W.H. Allen; 1968.

33. Bush TL. Noncontraceptive estrogen use and risk of cardiovascular disease: an overview and critique of the literature. In: Korenman SG, editor. The menopause: biological and clinical consequences of ovarian failure: evolution and management. Norwell (MA): Serono Symposia; 1990. p. 211–23.

34. Stampfer MJ, Colditz GA. Estrogen replacement therapy and coronary heart disease: a quantitative assessment of the epidemiologic evidence. Prev Med 1991; 20:47–63.

35. Grady D, Rubin SM, Petitti DB, et al. Hormone therapy to prevent disease and prolong life in postmenopausal women. Ann Intern Med 1992;117:1016–37.

36. Hulley S, Grady D, Bush T, et al. Randomized trial of estrogen plus progestin for secondary prevention of coronary heart disease in postmenopausal women. Heart and Estrogen/progestin Replacement Study (HERS) Research Group. JAMA 1998;280:605.

37. Grady D, Herrington D, Bittner V, et al, HERS research group. Cardiovascular disease outcomes during 6.8 years of hormone therapy: Heart and Estrogen/progestin Replacement Study follow-up (HERS II). JAMA 2002;288:49.

38. Hulley S, Furberg C, Barrett-Connor E, et al, HERS Research Group. Noncardiovascular disease outcomes during 6.8 years of hormone therapy: Heart and Estrogen/progestin Replacement Study follow-up (HERS II). JAMA 2002;288:58.

39. Manson JE, Hsia J, Johnson KC, et al, Women's Health Initiative Investigators. Estrogen plus progestin and the risk of coronary heart disease. N Engl J Med 2003; 349:523–34.

40. Anderson GL, Limacher M, Assaf AR, et al, Women's Health Initiative Steering Committee. Effects of conjugated equine estrogen in postmenopausal women with hysterectomy: the Women's Health Initiative randomized controlled trial. JAMA 2004;291:1701–12.

41. Sprague BL, Trentham-Dietz A, Cronin KA. A sustained decline in postmeno-pausal hormone use: results from the National Health and Nutrition Examination Survey, 1999-2010. Obstet Gynecol 2012;120:595.
42. Zouboulis CC, Makrantonaki E. Hormonal therapy of intrinsic aging. Rejuvenation Res 2012;15:302–12.
43. Samaras N, Samaras D, Frangos E, et al. A review of age-related dehydroepian-drosterone decline and its association with well-known geriatric syndromes: is treatment beneficial? Rejuvenation Res 2013;16:285–94.
44. Stuenkel CA, Davis SR, Gompel A, et al. Treatment of symptoms of the meno-pause: an Endocrine Society clinical practice guideline. J Clin Endocrinol Metab 2015;100:3975–4011.
45. Meeta, Digumarti L, Agarwal N, et al. Clinical practice guidelines on menopause: an executive summary and recommendations. J Midlife Health 2013;4:77–106.
46. Woods NF, Mitchell ES. Symptoms during the perimenopause: prevalence, severity, trajectory, and significance in women's lives. Am J Med 2005; 118(Suppl 12B):14–24.
47. Politi MC, Schleinitz MD, Col NF. Revisiting the duration of vasomotor symptoms of menopause: a meta-analysis. J Gen Intern Med 2008;23:1507–13.
48. Santen RJ, Allred DC, Ardoin SP, et al. Postmenopausal hormone therapy: an Endocrine Society scientific statement. J Clin Endocrinol Metab 2010;95:s1–66.
49. Barnabei VM, Cochrane BB, Aragaki AK, et al, Women's Health Initiative Investi-gators. Menopausal symptoms and treatment-related effects of estrogen and progestin in the Women's Health Initiative. Obstet Gynecol 2005;105(5 Pt 1): 1063–73.
50. Cardozo L, Bachmann G, McClish D, et al. Meta-analysis of estrogen therapy in the management of urogenital atrophy in postmenopausal women: second report of the hormones and urogenital therapy committee. Obstet Gynecol 1998;92: 722–7.
51. Management of symptomatic vulvovaginal atrophy: 2013 position statement of The North American Menopause Society. Menopause 2013;20:888–902.
52. Hays J, Ockene JK, Brunner RL, et al, Women's Health Initiative Investigators. Ef-fects of estrogen plus progestin on health-related quality of life. N Engl J Med 2003;348:1839.
53. Manson JE, Chlebowski RT, Stefanick ML, et al. Menopausal hormone therapy and health outcomes during the intervention and extended poststopping phases of the Women's Health Initiative randomized trials. JAMA 2013;310:1353–68.
54. Manson JE. Current recommendations: what is the clinician to do? Fertil Steril 2014 Apr;101(4):916–21.
55. Stone NJ, Robinson J, Lichtenstein AH, et al. 2013 ACC/AHA guideline on the treatment of blood cholesterol to reduce atherosclerotic cardiovascular risk in adults: a report of the American College of Cardiology/American Heart Associa-tion Task Force on Practice Guidelines. J Am Coll Cardiol 2014;63(25 Pt B): 2889–934.
56. Gleason CE, Dowling NM, Wharton W, et al. Effects of hormone therapy on cogni-tion and mood in recently postmenopausal women: findings from the random-ized, controlled KEEPS-cognitive and affective study. PLoS Med 2015;12(6): e1001833.
57. Chlebowski RT, Wactawski-Wende J, Ritenbaugh C, et al. Estrogen plus proges-tin and colorectal cancer in postmenopausal women. N Engl J Med 2004;350: 991–1004.

58. Anderson GL, Judd HL, Kaunitz AM, et al. Effects of estrogen plus progestin on gynecologic cancers and associated diagnostic procedures: the Women's Health Initiative randomized trial. JAMA 2003;290:1739–48.

59. Cauley JA, Robbins J, Chen Z, et al. Effects of estrogen plus progestin on risk of fracture and bone mineral density: the Women's Health Initiative randomized trial. JAMA 2003;290:1729–38.

60. Kanaya AM, Herrington D, Vittinghoff E, et al. Glycemic effects of postmenopausal hormone therapy: the Heart and Estrogen/progestin Replacement Study. A randomized, double-blind, placebo-controlled trial. Ann Intern Med 2003;138:1–9.

61. Margolis KL, Bonds DE, Rodabough RJ, et al. Effect of oestrogen plus progestin on the incidence of diabetes in postmenopausal women: results from the Women's Health Initiative Hormone Trial. Diabetologia 2004;47:1175–87.

62. Phillips TJ, Symons J, Menon S, et al. Does hormone therapy improve age-related skin changes in postmenopausal women? A randomized, double-blind, double-dummy, placebo-controlled multicenter study assessing the effects of norethindrone acetate and ethinyl estradiol in the improvement of mild to moderate age-related skin changes in postmenopausal women. J Am Acad Dermatol 2008;59:397–404.e3.

63. Rittié L, Kang S, Voorhees JJ, et al. Induction of collagen by estradiol: difference between sun-protected and photodamaged human skin in vivo. Arch Dermatol 2008;144:1129–40.

64. Maki PM, Gast MJ, Vieweg AJ, et al. Hormone therapy in menopausal women with cognitive complaints: a randomized, double-blind trial. Neurology 2007;69: 1322–30.

65. Espeland MA, Rapp SR, Shumaker SA, et al. Conjugated equine estrogens and global cognitive function in postmenopausal women: Women's Health Initiative Memory Study. JAMA 2004;291:2959–68.

66. Handelsman DJ. Trends and regional differences in testosterone prescribing in Australia, 1991-2001. Med J Aust 2004;181:419–22.

67. Basaria S. Reproductive aging in men. Endocrinol Metab Clin N Am 2013;42: 255–70.

68. Harman SM, Metter EJ, Tobin JD, et al. Longitudinal effects of aging on serum total and free testosterone levels in healthy men. J Clin Endocrinol Metab 2001;86: 724–31.

69. Araujo AB, Esche GR, Kupelian V, et al. Prevalence of symptomatic androgen deficiency in men. J Clin Endocrinol Metab 2007;92:4241–7.

70. Wu FC, Tajar A, Beynon JM, et al. Identification of late-onset hypogonadism in middle-aged and elderly men. N Engl J Med 2010;363:123–35.

71. Bhasin S, Cunningham GR, Hayes FJ, et al. Testosterone therapy in men with androgen deficiency syndromes: an Endocrine Society clinical practice guideline. J Clin Endocrinol Metab 2010;95:2536–59.

72. Boloña ER, Uraga MV, Haddad RY, et al. Testosterone use in men with sexual dysfunction: a systematic review and meta-analysis of randomized placebo-controlled trials. Mayo Clin Proc 2007;82:20–8.

73. Snyder PJ, Ellenberg SS, Cunningham GR, et al. The Testosterone Trials: Seven coordinated trials of testosterone treatment in elderly men. Clin Trials 2014;11: 362–75.

74. Gruenwald DA, Matsumoto AM. Testosterone supplementation therapy for older men: potential benefits and risks. J Am Geriatr Soc 2003;51:101–15.

75. Matsumoto AM. Testosterone administration in older men. Endocrinol Metab Clin N Am 2013;42:271–86.
76. Basaria S, Coviello AD, Travison TG, et al. Adverse events associated with testosterone administration. N Engl J Med 2010;363:109–22.
77. Mårin P, Holmäng S, Gustafsson C, et al. Androgen treatment of abdominally obese men. Obes Res 1993;1:245–51.
78. Snyder PJ, Peachey H, Hannoush P, et al. Effect of testosterone treatment on bone mineral density in men over 65 years of age. J Clin Endocrinol Metab 1999;84:1966–72.
79. English KM, Steeds RP, Jones TH, et al. Low-dose transdermal testosterone therapy improves angina threshold in men with chronic stable angina: a randomized, double-blind, placebo-controlled study. Circulation 2000;102:1906–11.
80. Kenny AM, Prestwood KM, Gruman CA, et al. Effects of transdermal testosterone on bone and muscle in older men with low bioavailable testosterone levels. J Gerontol A Biol Sci Med Sci 2001;56:M266–72.
81. Aversa A, Isidori AM, Spera G, et al. Androgens improve cavernous vasodilation and response to sildenafil in patients with erectile dysfunction. Clin Endocrinol 2003;58:632–8.
82. Steidle C, Schwartz S, Jacoby K, et al. AA2500 testosterone gel normalizes androgen levels in aging males with improvements in body composition and sexual function. J Clin Endocrinol Metab 2003;88:2673–81.
83. Shabsigh R, Kaufman JM, Steidel C, et al. Randomized study of testosterone gel as adjunctive therapy to sildenafil in hypogonadal men with erectile dysfunction who do not respond to sildenafil alone. J Urol 2004;172:658–63.
84. Seftel AD, Mack RJ, Secrest AR, et al. Restorative increases in serum testosterone levels are significantly correlated to improvements in sexual functioning. J Androl 2004;25:963–72.
85. Srinivas-Shankar U, Roberts SA, Connolly MJ, et al. Effects of testosterone on muscle strength, physical function, body composition, and quality of life in intermediate-frail and frail elderly men: a randomized, double-blind, placebo-controlled study. J Clin Endocrinol Metab 2010;95:639–50.
86. Cunningham GR, Stephens-Shields AJ, Rosen RC, et al. Testosterone treatment and sexual function in older men with low testosterone levels. J Clin Endocrinol Metab 2016;101:3096–104.
87. Roy CN, Snyder PJ, Stephens-Shields AJ, et al. Association of testosterone levels with anemia in older men: a controlled clinical trial. JAMA Intern Med 2017;177:480–90.
88. Resnick SM, Matsumoto AM, Stephens-Shields AJ, et al. Testosterone treatment and cognitive function in older men with low testosterone and age-associated memory impairment. JAMA 2017;317:717–27.
89. Budoff MJ, Ellenberg SS, Lewis CE, et al. Testosterone treatment and coronary artery plaque volume in older men with low testosterone. JAMA 2017;317:708–16.
90. Snyder PJ, Kopperdahl DL, Stephens-Shields AJ, et al. Effect of testosterone treatment on volumetric bone density and strength in older men with low testosterone: a controlled clinical trial. JAMA Intern Med 2017;177:471–9.

Depression in Older Adults

A Treatable Medical Condition

David A. Casey, MD

KEYWORDS

- Depression • Antidepressants • Electroconvulsive therapy

KEY POINTS

- Depression is not a normal part of the aging process.
- Depression in older adults is a treatable medical condition; a variety of psychotherapeutic and psychotherapeutic options are available.
- Electroconvulsive therapy is a useful treatment.
- The older patient must be viewed in their medical, functional, and social context for effective management.
- Cognition must be assessed along with mood in the older depressed patient.

INTRODUCTION

Depression is one of the most significant causes of emotional suffering in late life and may also be a contributing factor to the morbidity of many medical disorders.[1] Depressed elders often experience markedly diminished function and quality of life as well as mood symptoms. Increased mortality from both suicide and medical illness is also an important concomitant of depressive disorders in late life. Depression in older adults may be more persistent than depression earlier in life, often running a chronic, remitting course.[2] Clinical depression is not a part of normal aging but should be considered a treatable medical illness, although it certainly may be associated with problems of aging, such as loss, grief, and physical illness. The significance of late life depression is heightened by the fact that there are an increasing number of elders in the United States and many other countries.[3,4] The information in this article is particularly relevant to frail, medically ill, or cognitively impaired elders as well as the "old-old." The "old-old" is a somewhat ill-defined group, but here is used for those patients in their 80s or older. The use of age 65 as the onset of old age in geriatric medicine and psychiatry is arbitrary. Many such patients who are otherwise well may not require the specialized approach of the geriatrician.

Department of Psychiatry and Behavioral Sciences, Geriatric Psychiatry Program, University of Louisville School of Medicine, 401 East Chestnut Street, Suite 610, Louisville, KY 40202, USA
E-mail address: dacase01@exchange.louisville.edu

Prim Care Clin Office Pract 44 (2017) 499–510
http://dx.doi.org/10.1016/j.pop.2017.04.007
0095-4543/17/© 2017 Elsevier Inc. All rights reserved.

DIAGNOSTIC CONCEPTS

Major depression is the most significant form of depression recognized in the Diagnostic and Statistical Manual of Mental Disorders, 5th edition (DSM-5), the handbook of psychiatric diagnosis of the American Psychiatric Association used in the United States and elsewhere. DSM-5 defines major depression based on the presence of 5 or more core depressive symptoms during a 2-week period, including either depressed mood or loss of interest or pleasure, along with significant weight loss or gain (without dieting) or appetite change, insomnia or hypersomnia, psychomotor agitation or retardation, fatigue or loss of energy, feelings of worthlessness or inappropriate guilt, diminished ability to think or concentrate or indecisiveness, and recurrent thoughts of death or suicide.[5] No distinction is made in the DSM-5 depression criteria based on age or aging. One of the most significant and controversial changes in DSM-5 was the removal of the "bereavement exclusion." In DSM-IV and other earlier versions of the handbook, persons who had suffered a recent loss with grief reaction were excluded from the diagnosis of major depression. This change may affect older adults more than other groups.

In the past, some investigators regarded major depression as more common among the elderly than other groups. However, it now appears that the prevalence of major depression among those 65 years or older is approximately 1% to 4%, a prevalence similar to (or perhaps even lower than) other groups. However, some special groups of older adults have higher rates of depressive symptoms. Elders with chronic medical illnesses have rates of depression of about 25%, and nursing home residents have a prevalence of approximately 25% to 50%.[2,6–8]

"Minor depression" is another important concept in geriatric psychiatry. This condition is sometimes referred to as "subsyndromal or subthreshold depression." It is not a designated diagnostic category in DSM-5, but is denoted as a section under the category "other specified depressive disorders." It is usually described as having the presence of 1 of the 2 principal depressive symptoms plus 1 to 3 additional symptoms, although this definition is not universally accepted.[5] This condition appears to be common, although rates of minor depression differ widely in studies. Despite its name, minor depression is associated with levels of disability similar to that of major depression.[5,9,10]

Dysthymia (alternately known as persistent depressive disorder in DSM-5) is a chronic form of depression that is less severe than major depression and lasts 2 or more years.[5] Although it more commonly begins earlier in life, it may persist into old age.[11]

The overall prevalence of all clinically significant depressive symptoms among older adults has been estimated at 8% to 16%.[2] African American elders have been noted to have lower rates of depression and are less likely to take antidepressant medication.[12] Older women are more likely to be diagnosed with depression than are older men. Owing to this higher diagnosis rate as well as having a longer lifespan, most diagnosed elder depressives are women.

Age of onset is also an important concept in geriatric depression, with early and late life onset groups. Depressive disorders beginning earlier in life may be persistent or recurrent, continuing into old age. In early onset cases, depressive symptoms tend to be similar through the course of illness. Some new onset cases in late life may represent differences in cause, possibly based on brain aging or illness. An important example of late life onset illness is "vascular depression," thought to be related to cerebrovascular changes.[13,14] These patients seem to be more likely to have cognitive dysfunction (especially loss of executive function), along with reduced verbal fluency, psychomotor retardation, functional loss, and anhedonia. In addition, these patients seem to be less likely to have a family history of depression or psychotic symptoms.

Depression in late life often occurs in the context of multiple medical illnesses. Often, depressive symptoms are misattributed to the aging process itself or viewed as a normal response to loss or illness.[1] Older adult patients may also focus on the physical symptoms associated with a depressive illness, accompanied by minimization of the emotional aspects of the illness. The term "masked depression" has been used to describe this situation, although the use of this term has diminished owing to a lack of precision as a diagnostic concept.[15] Although stigma may have diminished somewhat over the past 2 decades, many elders still feel uncomfortable with any psychiatric label that they think stigmatizes them and may engage in self-stigmatization. Elderly patients who are clearly suffering from a depressive disorder may describe themselves as anxious or "feeling bad" rather than sad, a condition that has been referred to as "depression without sadness."[16] In the context of significant medical illness, depression may be overlooked. The DSM-5 approach to diagnosis by using specific criteria, which is designed to make diagnosis more objective, may occasionally become an obstacle in diagnosing older patients. The question of whether a particular symptom such as loss of energy or appetite "counts" toward the diagnosis of depression may be raised if a physical illness may potentially explain it. Geriatric psychiatrists commonly take the approach that a symptom should be counted if it is present, regardless of other possible explanations.[17]

The diagnosis of depression in older adults is also complicated by the presence of loss and grief. Obviously, such losses are a common part of aging, and grief following a major loss is normal.[1] However, the removal of the bereavement exclusion in DSM-5 was made because of the fact that loss or grief may trigger a clinically relevant depressive episode.

In addition to mood symptoms, older depressives may report preoccupation with bodily function (eg, constipation, pain, insomnia, or fatigue), multiple diffuse complaints, weight loss, anxiety, obsessional ruminations, difficulty making decisions, or marked negativity. Other symptoms may also include a preoccupation with finances, executive cognitive dysfunction, melancholia (lack of mood variation, social interactions, and psychomotor changes), and loss of function at a level similar to severe medical illness. Terms such as "failure to thrive" or "depletion syndrome" have sometimes been used to describe older depressed patients who have a combination of loss of appetite, weight loss, and marked apathy or loss of interest.[18,19] Elderly depressed patients as a group have much more significant functional loss than younger patients. Functional deficits may include such things as giving up activities, staying in bed, exaggerated helplessness, dependency, and extreme negativism. This loss of function with depression among older adults can be profound and disabling.

A depressive illness may sometimes be accompanied by delusions or hallucinations, a condition known as psychotic or delusional depression. Commonly, although not always, these psychotic symptoms have depressive themes. Illogical thinking may also occur. A syndrome known as catatonia may occasionally be associated with psychotic depression (in addition to other psychiatric or medical conditions such as bipolar disorder). Catatonia involves varying degrees of withdrawal and mutism, sometimes accompanied by rigidity. Rigidity may also be accompanied by a tendency to hold the limbs in unusual postures, particularly if placed there by an examiner (often described as waxy flexibility) or repeat or sustain illogical behaviors (stereotypy). Patients with psychotic depression may experience delusions of guilt, poverty, decay, or disease. Psychotic depression is common among depressed elderly inpatients, occurring in 20% to 45% of these patients. However, psychotic depression is much less common in outpatients. Treatment of psychotic depression may require a combination of an antipsychotic medication with an antidepressant. Electroconvulsive therapy (ECT) is thought to be the most effective therapy for this condition, especially if accompanied by catatonic symptoms.[20,21]

The role of genetics in late life depression is poorly understood. Although early life onset depression is often associated with a family history, this may not be the case with late life onset depression. No particular genetic risk factor in late life onset depression has been discovered.[22]

MEDICAL ILLNESS AND DEPRESSION

Medical illnesses commonly accompany depression in late life.[23] Stroke, diabetes, cancer, chronic lung disease, Alzheimer disease (AD), Parkinson disease, arthritis, and fractures are all associated with depressive symptoms or a depressive illness. Endocrine conditions such as hypothyroidism, aging-related changes in the adrenal axis, and reduced levels of testosterone may play a role in some cases. Weight loss is commonly associated with elder depression and may contribute to vulnerability to other medical conditions.[2,24,25] This interplay between depression and medical illness may be bidirectional. The interrelationship between ischemic heart disease and depression seems to be particularly important. Depression seems to contribute to the morbidity and mortality of certain cardiovascular conditions and may be a consequence of these illnesses as well.[26] However, it is not entirely clear that treatment with antidepressants will necessarily ameliorate these effects.[27] Some community studies show an association between depression in elders and overall mortality,[28] although associated factors such as smoking, chronic medical disease, and lack of social support may confound these observations. Depressed patients are also heavy consumers of medical care, and a disproportionate number of primary care visits for physical complaints are driven at least in part by depression.[29]

Many commonly prescribed medications used by elders may contribute to depressive symptoms. This list includes (among others) cancer/antineoplastic drugs, corticosteroids, antiparkinsonians, metoclopramide, interferon, and various cardiovascular and antihypertensive drugs. Of course, alcohol and other substances of abuse may contribute to depressive symptoms. A comprehensive review of the patient's medication list, including over-the-counter medications, is a necessary part of any evaluation of depression.[30] This review also considers factors of adherence. How the drug is actually taken (or not taken) is important to understand. Patients may take medicine originally prescribed for another person or for an earlier episode of illness. Factors of cost, accessibility, complexity of the regimen, and cognitive impairment may all impact adherence.

COGNITIVE SYMPTOMS AND DEPRESSION

Depression often has a negative impact on cognition, especially among older adults. Depression may even occasionally be misdiagnosed as a dementing illness. Some observers have suggested that depression with cognitive impairment may be a harbinger of incipient dementia (especially AD) as either a risk factor or an early indicator, even if the cognitive impairment improves as the depression is treated. Several recent studies lend credence to the view that depression, especially depression recurrent over a period of years, is associated with an increased risk of later developing dementia and AD.[31–33] The concept of "depressive pseudodementia,"[34] which was commonly used in the past, is no longer widely applied. It is now appreciated that the presence of both depressive and cognitive symptoms most commonly represents a mingling of disease processes rather than one illness masquerading as another. Frequently, depressive symptoms are observed in a person with an established diagnosis of dementia. The term "depression of Alzheimer's disease (AD)" has been proposed for patients who meet the diagnostic criteria for AD and also have at least 3 significant depressive symptoms (including depressed mood, anhedonia, poor appetite, poor sleep, social isolation, feelings of worthlessness, psychomotor changes, irritability, fatigue, and suicidal thoughts).[35]

SUICIDE IN OLDER ADULTS

Older adults in the United States have a high rate of suicide approximately double that of the general American population.[36] Although suicidal behaviors themselves do not seem to increase with advancing age, the rate of completed (successful) suicides increases dramatically. Men (especially whites) predominate in completed suicides among older adults. These elderly men typically select a highly lethal means of suicide, especially gunshot wound to the chest or head (instead of overdose or other less lethal means). African American elders, including men, seem to have a lower rate of suicide. Risk factors for elder suicide include the death of a spouse, living alone, poor perceived health, lack of a confidant, poor sleep, pain, hopelessness, access to a firearm, and other stressful life events. In many cases, elders who commit suicide have visited their primary care physician within a period of a few days before the event. It is therefore important for clinicians to inquire into the question of suicidal ideation. There is no evidence that doing so will awaken such ideas in patients.[36,37]

DIAGNOSTIC EVALUATION

Making the diagnosis of depression in the elderly is accomplished by clinical means, including interview, history, mental status examination, and collateral history. The use of depression scales such as the Patient Health Questionnaire-9, Geriatric Depression Scale, or Beck Depression Inventory may be highly useful to assist with diagnosis and also with tracking symptoms over time.[38,39] Physical and laboratory assessment is important to consider medical factors contributing to depressive symptoms. Laboratory evaluation is useful but often not conclusive, because there is no specific test or biomarker available at present. In many cases, there are multiple factors influencing depressive symptoms, including medical, social, and psychological components. Neuroimaging may be useful in some cases, especially if cerebrovascular disease, cognitive impairment, and dementia are considerations. The diagnostic evaluation should actively consider comorbid medical conditions as well as all medications (including over-the-counter medications). Assessment of cognitive status is also a necessary component of the overall evaluation. Once again, structured interview scales may be invaluable, such as the Montreal Cognitive Assessment, Saint Louis Mental Status, or Mini–Mental State Examination.[40–42] Functional status should include examination of gait and balance, nutritional status (including body weight and weight loss), and other activities of daily living.[24] The patient's living environment as well as family and social support should also be assessed.

TREATMENT OF DEPRESSION IN OLDER ADULTS

Depression in late life is a treatable condition and should be approached with the goal of achieving remission whenever possible. Up to 80% of patients recover from a depressive episode with appropriate therapy.[43] Successful treatment can lead to dramatic improvement in overall function and quality of life, especially in older adult patients. The degree of functional impairment in major depression in older adults is similar to that of a significant medical illness such as heart failure or chronic obstructive pulmonary disease. Treatments for depression include medication therapy, ECT, psychosocial therapies, as well as treatment of associated medical conditions. There is also support for physical activity[44] as well as (especially in seasonal depression) bright light therapy.[45] In regressed medically ill or catatonic patients, stimulants such as methylphenidate or amphetamine preparations may be helpful as stand-alone drugs or in combination with another antidepressant.[46] Stimulants require careful medical evaluation and monitoring. Despite concerns about the potential cardiovascular or psychotomimetic effects of stimulants, these very rarely occur. Instead, suppression of appetite and sleep disturbances are much more common issues. Despite aggressive therapy, however, depression may prove to be treatment resistant in some elders. Older adults are substantially more likely to suffer negative effects of psychiatric medications, which may also require a cautious approach.

There is no single preferred drug for depression in older adults, and a wide variety of medications may be used.[47,48] Selective serotonin reuptake inhibitors (SSRI) are often selected initially for older adults (especially citalopram, escitalopram, and sertraline).[2] Serotonin/norepinephrine reuptake inhibitors (SNRI) and other newer antidepressants (eg, mirtazapine, venlafaxine, desvenlafaxine, duloxetine, and bupropion) may also be used.[49] There is more limited clinical experience with the newest antidepressants with elderly patients (such as vortioxetine, vilazodone, and levomilnacipran). Tricyclic antidepressants and monoamine oxidase inhibitors are much less commonly used in the United States, because of a variety of side-effect and safety issues, but may still be helpful in treatment-resistant cases. The use of polypharmacy in depression has increased greatly, especially multiple antidepressants as well as antipsychotics. Despite these trends, geriatric specialists still seek to limit the number of medications for their patients.[49] In selected cases, antidepressant therapy may be augmented with atypical antipsychotics for agitated, psychotic, or treatment-resistant patients.[50] However, polypharmacy in older patients, especially frail patients, must be approached with an abundance of caution. It is also important to recognize that elders are often underrepresented in clinical trials of antidepressants, especially the types of physically ill, cognitively impaired, or frail patients often encountered in clinical settings.

Extra caution is required in dosing and monitoring for side effects (eg, sedation, ataxia, confusion, cardiovascular effects). The typical course of an antidepressant for an initial episode of major depression that responds to treatment is about 6 to 12 months. This course of treatment may be longer in cases of recurrent depression. Some patients require maintenance medication, especially those with chronic symptoms or frequent recurrences (especially more than 3 lifetime episodes). It may take 4 to 6 weeks to establish the efficacy of a particular antidepressant medication. Medication side effects are always a significant concern when treating elders. The SSRIs are generally regarded as the best tolerated antidepressants, but side effects may occur. They include drug-drug interactions (including cytochrome p-450 effects), hyponatremia, QT interval prolongation, and falling. Other possible side effects include weight loss, sexual dysfunction, agitation, gastrointestinal bleeding, serotonin syndrome, anticholinergic effects, and withdrawal effects.[2]

The response rate to an initial trial of a given antidepressant ranges from 50% to 65%, although there is a lack of data in this area specifically for older adult patients.[51] Multiple trials of medication may produce a higher response rate, although the rate of response to each new antidepressant trial falls after about 2 to 3 medication trials. Increasing the dose of medication beyond the typical level may be considered in cases where no side effects have occurred, especially if partial benefit has been observed. In the case of a treatment failure, a decision must be made whether to switch to a different medication, add a second antidepressant, or add another augmenting agent. Adding a second antidepressant is also often chosen when there is a partial response to the first drug. When adding a second antidepressant, an agent from a different pharmacologic class is usually selected. When switching to a new antidepressant, clinicians have historically also selected a drug from a new class. However, it now seems clear that even when a drug from a particular class has failed, the likelihood of success with a drug from the same class or a different class is about equal. Historically, buspirone, thyroid medications, and lithium were among the typical selections for augmentation. However, today it is more common to add an atypical antipsychotic such as aripiprazole or quetiapine, typically in low doses. If polypharmacy is considered, the potential harmful effects must be weighed against the possibility of boosting response rate. Some common mistakes in antidepressant therapy include reliance on antianxiety or sleeping medications (especially benzodiazepines), excessive polypharmacy, inadequate dose or duration of medication trial, and giving up too soon. Genomic testing for antidepressants has recently been made available, attempting to screen patients for any genetic condition that might have an impact on the utility or side-effect profile of several different medications. However, the clinical utility of this approach, especially in older patients, is not yet clear.

Anxiety symptoms and disorders commonly cooccur with depression among elderly patients. In the past, benzodiazepines or other sedative hypnotics have been widely prescribed. However, an abundance of evidence is now available highlighting the potential risks of benzodiazepines and related medications. These risks include sedation, falling, accidents, cognitive clouding, increased risk of developing dementia, and others. The use of benzodiazepines should be limited. A common clinical dilemma is the case of a depressed or anxious older adult patient who has been taking a benzodiazepine for several years at the time of evaluation. Such a patient is very likely to have both physical and psychological dependence on the medication and be very reluctant to discontinue it. The best approach is usually to establish a strong therapeutic alliance with the patient, reassure them that their concerns are important, seek to address the symptoms in alternate ways, and very gradually wean the medication over a period of months.

ELECTROCONVULSIVE THERAPY

ECT can be used safely and effectively in elders for severe or treatment-resistant depression, despite the controversies that have existed about this treatment over a period of decades.[52,53] Treatment resistance in this case may be defined as a failure of at least 2 well-conducted trials of medication therapy. A very large number of older patients would be classified into this category, but in clinical practice, only the most severe cases are generally considered for ECT. Another group of good candidates for ECT includes those patients who have responded well to ECT in the past. In such cases, it is often prudent to consider ECT early in the course of a relapse rather than waiting for multiple medication failures. ECT typically involves a series of roughly 6 to 12 treatments over a period of several weeks, although the number of treatments is determined by the patient's response. ECT may sometimes be effective in treatment-resistant cases of depression even when multiple medications have failed. The overall response rate in ECT is much higher than with medications, in the 80% to 90% range. ECT is the treatment of choice for most patients with catatonia and is also a highly effective therapy for psychotic depression. Relative to medications, it has a much more rapid rate of response. Despite these relative advantages, ECT is not a permanent cure for depression. It is best regarded as a potent treatment of a given episode. It also has several drawbacks, including the need for general anesthesia, and the risk of short-term cognitive impairment. Although ECT may sometimes be conducted on an outpatient basis, many elders with medical or frailty issues require psychiatric hospitalization for the treatment. Despite substantial literature on ECT in the elderly, there are very few rigorous studies, and ECT does not lend itself to placebo controlled trials, the gold standard of outcome measures.[54] Nevertheless, the available evidence strongly suggests that ECT for elders has an excellent safety and effectiveness record, especially considering the consequences of unremitting depression. In selected patients, maintenance ECT may be advisable to maintain a state of remission. Maintenance ECT is usually considered in cases where there is an established tendency toward rapid relapse into depression. Occasionally, ECT may be used in other conditions, including mania and catatonic syndromes not clearly associated with depression (such as neuroleptic malignant syndrome, Parkinson disease, or dementia). Alternatives to ECT have been introduced in recent years, including repetitive transcranial stimulation (rTMS). rTMS is a therapy for treatment-resistant depression involving repetitively stimulating a portion of the frontal cortex with a powerful magnetic coil. The treatment is performed on an outpatient basis over a period of weeks, typically involving roughly 25 to 30 sessions. No anesthesia is required; no seizure is induced, and there is no cognitive impairment associated with the therapy. The overall success rates for this treatment are lower than for ECT (for all patients, about 50%–60%), although patient acceptance and tolerance are high. The long-term effects of rTMS on the course of depression are not yet clear. Experience with rTMS for elders so far is somewhat limited, and the results appear to be mixed with a suggestion that elders as a group may not respond as well as younger patients.[55]

PSYCHOSOCIAL THERAPIES

A variety of psychological factors may play a role in elder depression. These psychological issues may include grief and loss, widowhood, the "empty nest," retirement, pain, and illness. Regrets experienced over a lifetime may play a role in an older patient. Fears of financial problems, dependency, loneliness, existential issues of aging, and mortality are also potent issues. A belief once existed that older adult patients were not suitable candidates for psychotherapy. Experience has shown that a variety of approaches that have been developed for late life psychotherapy may be helpful for depression. Supportive psychotherapy focuses on ego support, practical advice, medication compliance, psychoeducation, activities, and maintaining a hopeful attitude. Cognitive behavioral therapy (CBT) is a structured, agenda-based therapy focusing on identifying and modifying self-defeating patterns of thought and behavior in the present, rather than focusing on the unconscious or the distant past.[56,57] The patient is encouraged to acquire skills in therapy that may be useful in addressing depressive symptoms directly and serve to limit the risk of relapse. Modifications of CBT may be required, especially for the frail, physically ill, or cognitively impaired older adult patient.[58,59] The therapist may need to adapt the pace and process of therapy in the case of loss of attention, stamina, and slowed thinking. The therapist may have to be more active and provide sufficient energy to engage the elderly patient. The family often needs to be involved to a greater extent than in nongeriatric patients. The typical here-and-now focus of CBT may be relaxed to allow for life review and existential tasks. Homework assignments, a typical element of CBT, may be simple and immediate. Aspects of CBT with elders may include behavioral activation, positive reinforcement, identifying strengths, and realistic coping with loss or illness.

Interpersonal therapy involves a focus on roles and role transitions and has been much discussed but little used in older depressive outside of academic centers.[60] Problem-solving therapy is a relatively new and promising therapy that focuses on helping depressed patients recognize key life problems and develop and implement practical plans to address them.[61,62]

BIPOLAR DEPRESSION IN OLDER ADULTS

Bipolar disorder typically has its onset in the late adolescent or young adult years. However, the disorder is a life-long condition of remitting and relapsing episodes of mood disorder. Bipolar disorder is unfortunately associated with a high level of mortality and a shortened lifespan by up to 2 decades in the United States. Nevertheless, although younger patients are more commonly discussed in the literature, older patients with bipolar depression are relatively frequently encountered in geriatric practice. There are few guidelines for treating these patients. They may present with mixed or irritable symptoms or episodes rather than the typical highs or lows, and well or euthymic periods may be briefer. Cognitive impairment and a high degree of medical morbidity appear to be common in this population. Psychotic depression and catatonia also appear to be overrepresented. The usual mood stabilizers may be useful, such as divalproex, carbamazepine, and lithium, but may be more difficult to manage and may require lower doses and blood levels. Anecdotal evidence suggests that antidepressants are more commonly used in this group than in younger bipolars, and may be better tolerated.

SUMMARY

Depression is not a normal part of aging and should be regarded as a serious, disabling medical disorder. There are a growing number of cases of late life depression owing to a growth in the at-risk population, although an earlier belief that depression increases with age appears to be incorrect. The prevalence of depression in older American adults appears to be similar to other age groups. A major focus of the field is to understand how depression among older adults intersects with grief, medical illnesses, and dementia. The illness is recognized as heterogeneous, and various diagnostic constructs may be applied. These constructs include major depression, minor depression, persistent depressive disorder, late life onset depression, vascular depression, and depression of AD, among others. Suicide is an important consideration in the management of elder depression, especially among older white men; an active approach by clinicians is warranted. Pharmacotherapy is important, especially with the SSRIs and SNRIs. ECT remains an important option, especially for catatonic, psychotic, or treatment-resistant cases of elder depression, but the role of rTMS is still being clarified. Psychotherapy is an important and often overlooked treatment option for geriatric depression, and our knowledge in this area has grown greatly in recent years, particularly for CBT. Depression in the elderly should be viewed as a treatable condition. Successful treatment may greatly improve the patient's function and quality of life.

REFERENCES

1. Casey DA. Depression in the elderly: a review and update. Asia Pac Psychiatr 2011;4:160–7.
2. Blazer D. Depression in late life: review and commentary. Focus 2009;7:118–36 [reprinted from J Gerontol A Biol Sci Med Sci 2003;58A(3):249–65].

3. Alexopolous GS, Kelly RE. Research advances in geriatric depression. World Psychiatry 2009;8(3):140–9.
4. Day JC. U.S. Bureau of the Census: population projections in the United States, by age, sex, race, and Hispanic origin, 1993-2050. Current population reports. Washington, DC: U.S. Government Printing Office; 1996. p. 25–1104.
5. American Psychiatric Association: Diagnostic and Statistical Manual of Mental Disorders (DSM-5). 5th Edition. Arlington (VA): American Psychiatric Association; 2013. p. 160–8.
6. Steffens DC, Skoog I, Norton MC, et al. Prevalence of depression and its treatment in an elderly population. Arch Gen Psychiatry 2000;57:601–7.
7. Yohannes AM, Baldwin RC, Connolly MJ. Prevalence of depression and anxiety symptoms in elderly patients admitted in post-acute intermediate care. Int J Geriatr Psychiatry 2008;23:1141–7.
8. Jongenelis K, Pot AM, Eisses AM, et al. Prevalence and risk indicators of depression in elderly nursing home patients: the AGED study. J Affect Disord 2004; 83(2–3):135–42.
9. Lyness JM, Heo M, Datto CJ, et al. Outcomes of minor and subsyndromal depression among elderly patients in primary care settings. Ann Intern Med 2006;144:496–504.
10. Vahia IV, Meeks TW, Thompson WK, et al. Subthreshold depression and successful aging in older women. Am J Geriatr Psychiatry 2010;18(3):212–20.
11. Williams JW, Barrett J, Oxman T, et al. Treatment of dysthymia and minor depression in primary care. J Am Med Assoc 2000;284(12):1519–26.
12. Cohen CI, Magai C, Yaffee R, et al. Racial differences in syndromal and subsyndromal depression in an older urban population. Psychiatr Serv 2005;56(12): 1556–63.
13. Alexopolous GS. The vascular depression hypothesis: 10 years later. Biol Psychiatry 2006;60:1304–5.
14. Sneed JR, Culang-Reinlieb ME. The vascular depression hypothesis: an update. Am J Geriatr Psychiatry 2011;19(2):99–103.
15. Beck AT, Alford BA. Depression: causes and treatment. 2nd edition. Philadelphia: University of Pennsylvania Press; 2009. p. 77.
16. Gallo JJ, Rabins PV. Depression without sadness: alternative presentations of depression in late life. Am Fam Physician 1999;60:820–6.
17. Evans M, Mottram P. Diagnosis of depression in elderly patients. Adv Psychiatr Treat 2000;6:49–56.
18. Robertson RG, Montagnini M. Geriatric failure to thrive. Am Fam Physician 2004; 70(2):343–50.
19. Adams KB. Depressive symptoms, depletion, or developmental change? Withdrawal, apathy, and lack of vigor on the geriatric depression scale. Gerontologist 2001;41(6):768–77.
20. Kennedy G. Advances in the treatment of late-life psychotic depression. Prim Psychiatr 2004;15(7):27–9.
21. Meyers BS, Flint AJ, Rothschild AJ, et al. A double-blind randomized controlled trial of olanzapine plus sertraline vs olanzapine plus placebo for psychotic depression. Arch Gen Psychiatry 2009;66(8):838–47.
22. Steffens DC. Imaging and genetics advances in understanding geriatric depression. Neuropsychopharmacology 2010;35:348–9.
23. Casey DA. Management of the patient in geriatric psychiatry. In: Tasman A, Kay J, Lieberman J, et al, editors. Psychiatry. 3rd edition. Chichester (England): Wiley; 2008. p. 2549–62.

24. Charlson M, Peterson JC. Medical comorbidity and late life depression: what is known and what are the unmet needs? Biol Psychiatry 2002;52:226–35.
25. Noel PH, Williams JW, Unutzer J, et al. Depression and comorbid illness in elderly primary care patients: impact on multiple domains of health status and well-being. Ann Fam Med 2004;2(6):555–62.
26. Bigger JT, Glassman AH. The American Heart Association science advisory on depression and coronary heart disease: an exploration of the issues raised. Cleve Clin J Med 2010;77(Suppl 3):S12–9.
27. Pitt B, Deldin PJ. Depression and cardiovascular disease: have a happy day-just smile! Eur Heart J 2010;31(9):1036–7.
28. Cho HJ, Lavretsky H, Olmstead R, et al. Prior depression history and deterioration of physical health in community-dwelling older adults-a prospective cohort study. Am J Geriatr Psychiatry 2010;18(5):442–51.
29. Luber MP, Meyers BS, Williams-Russo PG, et al. Depression and service utilization in elderly primary care patients. Am J Geriatr Psychiatry 2001;9(2):169–76.
30. Dhondt T, Beekman AT, Deeg DJ, et al. Iatrogenic depression in the elderly: results from a community based study in the Netherlands. Soc Psychiatry Psychiatr Epidemiol 2002;37(8):393–8.
31. Beal E. Dementia: depression and dementia. Nat Rev Neurol 2010;6(9):470.
32. Dotson VM, Beydoun MA, Zonderman AB. Recurrent depressive symptoms and the incidence of dementia and mild cognitive impairment. Neurology 2010;75:27–34.
33. Saczynski JS, Beiser A, Seshadri S, et al. Depressive symptoms and risk of dementia. Neurology 2010;75:35–41.
34. Wells CE. Pseudodementia. Am J Psychiatry 1979;136:895–900.
35. Rosenberg PB, Onyike C, Katz IR, et al. Clinical application of operationalized criteria for "Depression of Alzheimer's disease". Int J Geriatr Psychiatry 2005;20(2):119–27.
36. Casey DA. Suicide in the elderly: a two-year study of data from death certificates. South Med J 1991;84(10):1185–7.
37. Conwell Y, Thompson C. Suicidal behavior in elders. Psychiatr Clin North Am 2008;31(2):333–56.
38. Yesavage JA, Brink TL, Rose TL, et al. Development and validation of a geriatric depression screening scale: a preliminary report. J Psychiatr Res 1982–1983;17(1):37–49.
39. Phelan E, Williams B, Meeker K, et al. A study of the diagnostic accuracy of the PHQ-9 in primary care elderly. BMC Fam Pract 2010;11:63.
40. Folstein MF, Folstein SE, McHugh PR. "Mini-mental state": a practical method for grading the cognitive state of patients for the clinician. J Psychiatr Res 1975;12(3):189–98.
41. Nasreddine ZS, Phillips NA, Bedirian V, et al. The Montreal Cognitive Assessment, MoCA: a brief screening tool for mild cognitive impairment. J Am Geriatr Soc 2005;53(4):695–9.
42. Tariq SH, Tumosa N, Chibnall JT, et al. Comparison of the Saint Louis University mental status examination and the mini-mental state examination for detecting dementia and mild neurocognitive disorder-a pilot study. Am J Geriatr Psychiatry 2006;14(11):900–10.
43. Reynolds E, Frank C, Perel J, et al. Combined pharmacotherapy and psychotherapy in the acute and continuation treatment of elderly patients with recurrent major depression: a preliminary report. Am J Psychiatry 1992;149:1687–92.

44. Sjoesten N, Kivel SL. The effects of physical exercise on depressive symptoms among the aged: a systematic review. Int J Geriatr Psychiatry 2006;21(5):410–8.

45. Lieverse R, Van Someren EJ, Nielen MM, et al. Bright light treatment in elderly patients with non-seasonal major depressive disorder. A randomized placebo controlled trial. Arch Gen Psychiatry 2011;68(1):61–70.

46. Prowler ML, Weiss D, Caroff SN. Treatment of catatonia with methylphenidate in an elderly patient with depression. Psychosomatics 2010;51(1):74–6.

47. Salzman C, Wong E, Wright BC. Drug and ECT treatment of depression in the elderly, 1996-2001: a literature review. Biol Psychiatry 2002;52(3):265–84.

48. Alexopoulos GS. Depression in the elderly. Lancet 2005;365(9475):1961–70.

49. Alexopoulos GS, Katz IR, Reynolds CF, et al. The expert consensus guideline series. Pharmacotherapy of depressive disorders in older patients. Postgrad Med 2001;Spec No Pharmacotherapy: special edition:1–86.

50. Alexopoulos GS. Pharmacotherapy for late-life depression. J Clin Psychiatry 2011;72(1):e04.

51. Taylor WD, Doraiswamy PM. A systematic review of antidepressant placebo-controlled trials for geriatric depression: limitations of current data and directions for the future. Neuropsychopharmacology 2004;29:2285–99.

52. Casey DA, Davis MH. Electroconvulsive therapy in the very old. Gen Hosp Psychiatry 1996;18:436–9.

53. Flint AJ, Gagnon N. Effective use of electroconvulsive therapy in late-life depression. Can J Psychiatry 2002;47(8):734–41.

54. van der Wurff FB, Stek ML, Hoogendijk WJ, et al. The efficacy and safety of ECT in depressed older adults, a literature review. Int J Geriatr Psychiatry 2003;18:894–904.

55. Jalenques I, Legrand G, Vaille-Perret E, et al. Therapeutic efficacy and safety of repetitive transcranial magnetic stimulation in depressions of the elderly: a review. Encephale 2009;36(Suppl 2):D105–18 [in French].

56. Laidlaw K, Thompson LW, Gallagher-Thompson D, et al. Cognitive behaviour therapy with older people. West Sussex (United Kingdom): Wiley; 2003. p. 232.

57. Gallagher-Thompson D, Thompson LW. Treating later life depression. A cognitive-behavioral approach, therapist guide. New York: Oxford University Press; 2010. p. 241.

58. Evans C. Cognitive-behavioural therapy with older people. Adv Psychiatr Treat 2007;13(2):111–8.

59. Casey DA, Grant RW. Cognitive therapy with geropsychiatric inpatients. In: Wright JH, Thase ME, Beck AT, et al, editors. The cognitive milieu: inpatient applications of cognitive therapy. New York: Guilford Publications; 1992. p. 295–314.

60. Miller MD. Using interpersonal therapy (IPT) with older adults today and tomorrow: a review of the literature and new developments. Curr Psychiatry Rep 2008;10(1):16–22.

61. Alexopoulos GS, Raue P, Arean P. Problem-solving therapy vs. supportive therapy in geriatric major depression with executive dysfunction. Am J Geriatr Psychiatry 2003;11(1):46–52.

62. Arean P, Raue P, Mackin RS, et al. Problem solving therapy and supportive therapy for older adults with major depression and executive dysfunction. Am J Psychiatry 2010;167(11):1391–8.

Advance Care Planning in the Outpatient Geriatric Medicine Setting

Bryan David Struck, MD[a,b,]*, Elizabeth Aubrey Brown, MD[b,c],
Stefani Madison, MD[d]

KEYWORDS

- Advance care planning • Geriatric medicine clinic • Advance directive • POLST

KEY POINTS

- Advance care planning contributes to patient-centered care in the outpatient geriatric medicine clinic.
- Advance care planning can include advance directives, Physician Orders for Life Sustaining Treatment (POLST), and do-not-resuscitate orders.
- Leading advance care planning conversations requires skill, which can be developed over time.
- Medicare allows for advance care planning conversations to be reimbursed if documented correctly.

Patient-centered care is the new mantra for health care. The concept is simple, defined as "care that is respectful of and responsive to individual patient preferences, needs, and values and [ensures] that patient values guide all clinical decisions."[1] This type of care is the cornerstone of geriatric medicine. Geriatric patients have complex medical needs and often must make complex decisions regarding specific treatments and the impact of treatments on their future health. Advance care planning provides the method to ensure that patient values guide clinical decision making. Advance care planning involves discussing future medical decisions that a patient might need to make, letting others know about their preferences, and documenting those preferences in an advance directive.[2] This article discusses how advance care planning can be done effectively and efficiently in the outpatient geriatric medicine setting.

Geriatric patients live with chronic illness that can have significant impacts on their health. Approximately 60% of older adults live with 2 or more chronic illnesses, such

[a] Hospice and Palliative Care Medicine, Oklahoma City VA Medical Center, 921 NE 13th 11G, Oklahoma City, OK 73104, USA; [b] Reynolds Department of Geriatric Medicine, University of Oklahoma Health Sciences Center, 1122 NE 13th ORB 1200, Oklahoma City, OK 73117, USA; [c] Oklahoma City VA Medical Center, 921 NE 13th 11G, Oklahoma City, OK 73104, USA; [d] Denver Health, Davis Pavilion (Pavilion E) 700, Delaware Street, Denver, CO 80204, USA
* Corresponding author. Hospice and Palliative Care Medicine, Oklahoma City VA Medical Center, Oklahoma City, OK.
E-mail address: Bryan.struck@VA.gov

Prim Care Clin Office Pract 44 (2017) 511–518
http://dx.doi.org/10.1016/j.pop.2017.04.008
0095-4543/17/Published by Elsevier Inc.
primarycare.theclinics.com

as heart disease, chronic obstructive pulmonary disease, stroke, diabetes, cancer, and dementia.[3] These illnesses are common causes of death in the adult population. As a result, advance care planning is very important to geriatric patients. However, 70% of adults 65 years of age or older have completed some type of advance care planning,[4] although this completion rate varies among patient demographics and clinical settings. The 1990 Patient Self Determination Act requires hospitals and skilled nursing facilities to ask each patient on admission whether they have an advance directive and, if present, to record it in the patient's medical record.[5] The law does not require a patient to complete an advance directive for treatment. The law requires individual states to determine how the advance directive is written and implemented, resulting in variation from state to state. The basic components of an advance directive include (1) identification of a health care proxy, (2) how future care should be done when faced with a terminal or end-stage illness, and (3) ability to document a do-not-resuscitate order if desired. These basic components of the advance directive should be honored when a patient crosses state lines. A state advance directive should be honored if a patient seeks care in a federal facility such as a Veterans' Affairs (VA) medical center. However, if the advance directive discusses components that are noncompliant with local state laws (such as states with death-with-dignity laws or assisted-death laws), these components would not be honored. The geriatric clinic must have a firm knowledge of the state laws regarding advance directives and advance care planning.

Geriatric assessment offers many assessment tools that focus on function, cognition, and polypharmacy. Advance care planning should be included in this discussion. Somewhere between social history and activities of daily living, the clinician should ask whether the patient has an advance directive. If the patient has, a directive, the clinician should ask for the advance directive to be brought to the office so that it may be added to the electronic medical record. Geriatric patients may have opportunities to complete an advance directive outside of a clinic or hospital. These sites may include churches, senior centers, or an attorney's office. Patients completing advance directives at these sites may not have discussed the document with health care personnel and may need to review the document for clarity in the clinic. A patient's formal estate planning or trust may include advance care planning. If a patient has only completed a will, advance care planning would not be included. Other excellent opportunities to discuss advance directives and advance care planning include after hospitalization for exacerbation of chronic illness, after a new diagnosis of serious illness, or when moving to a new place because activities of daily living or instrumental activities of daily living have become impaired.

Advance care planning conversations have shown great benefit in decreasing hospitalizations, decreasing intensive treatments at end of life, increasing hospice use, and ensuring that patients die in the environment of their choice.[4] These benefits lead to cost-effective and high-quality treatment at end of life.[6] As a result, Medicare recognizes the importance of these conversations and developed Centers for Medicare & Medicaid Services codes for reimbursement after these conversations have been held.[7]

- CPT (Current Procedural Terminology) code 99497: advance care planning including the explanation and discussion of advance directives such as standard forms (with completion of such forms, when performed) by the physician or other qualified health care professional; first 30 minutes, face to face with the patient, family members, and/or surrogate

- CPT code 99498: each additional 30 minutes (list separately in addition to code for primary procedure)

The codes used to bill for advance care planning conversations are time based. Under Medicare guidelines, clinicians must spend at least 30 minutes performing the advance care planning service otherwise they should consider billing a different evaluation and management service. The service can be billed on the same day as other evaluation and management services, transitional care management services, or chronic care management services. This service can be performed in any location and billed appropriately.

These conversations are held by physicians or other qualified health professionals, face to face with patient, family, and/or the surrogate decision maker. In a team-based approach, nonphysician practitioners and other staff under the supervision and direction of a treating physician can perform the services. There are no limits on the number of times advance care planning can be reported in any given time period. However, a reasonable cause for repeat discussions should be documented. Changes in a patient's health status or discussing wishes regarding end-of-life care are common reasons for the service being billed multiple times. The advance care planning conversation is paid for by Medicare part B when it is medically necessary. Advance care planning is an optional element of the annual wellness visit. If billed as part of the annual wellness visit, the advance care planning discussion must be held on the same day as the annual wellness visit, be held by the same provider as the annual wellness visit, and be coded with the modifier 33. In addition, when part of the wellness examination, the advance care planning discussion is not subject to the Medicare part B deduction and coinsurance. Note that the service is elective, and patients should be given the opportunity to decline the services.

To properly document this conversation, you should include an account of the conversation, the parties included in the conversation (ie, patient, family members, and/or surrogate decision makers), what forms were discussed and the extent of explanation, and how much time was spent face to face. Completing an advance directive or other advance care planning document is not necessary to bill under the services. It is also recommended to include the diagnosis and ICD-10 (International Classification of Diseases, 10th Revision) code, which is used to guide the discussion unless the advance care planning conversation is part of the wellness examination.

As patient-centered care propels advance care planning to the forefront of quality medicine, clinicians must ensure that all health care personnel can perform these conversations with expertise. Leading advance care planning discussion is a skill that can be developed and improved as clinicians practice medicine. These conversations must be done with skill because geriatric patients may be reluctant to discuss advance care planning because they are concerned the conversation may mean that something bad will happen or the conversations will lead to unwanted changes in treatment. In the past, medical education followed the construct that physicians would learn to do these conversations as they went along. That mindset is now changing. Googling "advance care planning conversation" or "goals of care conversation" will find multiple Web sites showing how-to algorithms for conducting these conversations and courses that teach clinicians how to improve this skill. Resources for skill improvement include:

1. Reading narratives such as *Being Mortal* by Atul Gawande[8]
2. Following a protocol such as SPIKES (Setup, Perception, Invitation, Knowledge, Emotion, Summarize/Strategize) for goals of care discussion[9,10]
3. Enrolling in a skill workshop presented at annual meetings from the American Academy of Hospice and Palliative Medicine, American Academy of Family Physicians, or American Geriatrics Society

The VA's National Center for Ethics in Health Care provides a curriculum entitled Goals of Care Conversations Training for Physicians, Advance Practice Registered

Nurses, and Physician Assistants. Clinician educators may use this curriculum to conduct face-to-face sessions in which participants actively practice communication skills.[11] If these conversations are done poorly, miscommunication and dissatisfaction with the health care system may occur. If these conversations are done effectively, the patient-doctor relationship can grow stronger and the patient values are allowed to determine care.

To begin this conversation, rapport must be established with the older adult. This rapport is very important if the discussion is occurring during the first clinical encounter in the geriatric clinic. To build rapport, explore what patients do for enjoyment, explore their support networks, explore what they want to accomplish with the visits, explore what concerns them about their current illnesses, and explore what brings meaning to their lives. Although these questions may seem to be unimportant in a clinic with time restrictions, they provide a wealth of information about the values that will form the patient's clinical decision making. Once there is an understanding about the patient as a person, the clinician can begin the discussion by normalizing the advance care planning conversation. Possible ways to normalize the conversation include telling the patient that anyone more than 18 years old should have an advance directive or that advance care planning is important for anyone with chronic serious illness. If applicable, explain how state laws affect their health care if they do not participate in advance care planning. Before proceeding to the "Do you want to be resuscitated?" question, begin with a less serious question such as, "Do you know who want to speak on your behalf if you are unable speak to your physician and health care team for any reason?."

Once the conversation is started, it is important for the patient to understand why the physician or health care team has decided to have this conversation. Reasons include that the illness is progressing, the serious illness is being affected by other chronic illnesses (synergistic effect), or that a new diagnosis will have a major impact on the patient's health. If the patient is reluctant to begin the conversation, explore where the reluctance originates. **Box 1** offers scripts for introducing advance care planning when there are changes in the clinical condition.[12] Possible barriers include denial of severity of illness, the patient's experience with loved ones who had similar conversations that resulted in a perceived negative outcome, and not wanting to have the conversation without the support system present. Patients may believe that, if they have this conversation, they are giving up hope. Geriatric patients value independence, preserved function, and preserved cognition. These values may play a significant role in the patient's medical decisions and should be included in advance care planning conversations. Patients may be more concerned about the impact of an illness or treatment limiting their ability to continue to live independently or causing further decline in their health without providing real benefit. These concerns may be present for geriatric patients deciding on treatments with significant impacts on health, such as chemotherapy, dialysis, or high-risk cardiac procedures. If a treatment does not support the patient's values or goals, then an alternative plan of care should be developed with input from the patient and the health care team.

Ideally the advance care planning conversation should occur early, before there is a medical crisis. Although this conversation is important, patients may not be ready to have it at this clinical encounter and should not be pressured into having the conversation. However, reluctance to have the conversation should not imply that it should never be brought up again. It is important to assure patients that it is acceptable to have this conversation with their families or proxies before making decisions. At future visits, the physician or health care team should remind the patient that the conversation was started in the past and inquire whether they are ready to continue the

---

Box 1
Scripts for introducing advance care planning

Routine visit with no recent changes in health status

It looks like you are doing well right now, and I expect it to continue that way in the near future. I like to talk with all my patients about their preferences for care in case they get very sick and to determine who they would want to make decisions for them if they were too sick to make their own decisions. I think it's best to talk about these things when patients are feeling well and long before we have to react to a crisis. That gives both of us plenty of time to talk about what matters to you so that I can give you the kinds of care that match your goals. Would it be okay for us to talk about this today?

Episode of acute illness or hospitalization

To make sure that we are working together while you are so sick, it is important that we talk about your goals for care at this time. I know it can be hard to think about these things when you are ill, but would it be okay for us to spend a little time talking about this right now?

Follow-up visit after illness exacerbation

You were pretty sick last time I saw you. Are you feeling better now? It's at times like this that I like to talk about goals of care to make sure that I'm up to date with what you would want in case you have another episode like that and others might have to make decisions for you. Would it be okay for us to talk about this now?

From Starks H, Vig EK, Pearlman RA. Advance care planning. In: Palliative care core skills and clinical competencies. 2nd edition. Philadelphia: Elsevier Saunders; 2011. (Box 20-1); with permission.

---

conversation. **Box 2** summarizes the steps that can be taken for effective advance care planning conversations in the geriatric clinic.

As the advance care planning discussions continue, geriatric patients may be ready to definitively document in writing their specific plans for end-of-life care and go beyond what is indicated in an advance directive. The patient may choose to complete an out-of-hospital do-not-resuscitate order. Care must be taken to ensure that the patient understands that, with this order, no resuscitation attempt will be made. If this order must be rescinded for specific treatments (eg, hip fracture fixation), the patient must determine when the order is to be reinstated and communicate this to the health care team.

Another option for documenting specific plans is to use the Physician Orders for Life Sustaining Treatment (POLST).[13,14] The POLST is a portable medical order documenting the patient's wishes. These orders were developed in Oregon in 1991 as a way to focus on improving medical care in individuals with a serious illness or frailty at the end of life. However, an advance directive is not sufficient to ensure that the patient's end-of-life wishes are honored. Because the advance directive may be completed far in advance of a serious illness diagnosis, the advance directive may not provide enough information to help with medical decision making in all clinical situations. The POLST paradigm was created using evidence-based medicine to create a best-practices model and, just as advance care planning is voluntary, completing a POLST is also voluntary.

POLST is also known by the following acronyms:

- MOLST (Medical Orders for Life-Sustaining Treatment)
- MOST (Medical Orders for Scope of Treatment)

Box 2
Seven steps for effective advance care planning conversations in the geriatric clinic

1. Build rapport: learn about geriatric patients as people, not just as sets of chronic illnesses.

2. Normalize the conversation: let geriatric patients know that everyone more than 18 years of age needs this discussion.

3. Know your state laws regarding advance directives, advance care planning, and Physician Orders for Life Sustaining Treatment. Inform patients how the laws affect their health decisions and treatments.

4. Begin with a nonserious question by asking geriatric patients who they want to speak on their behalf if they are unable speak to their physicians and health care teams for any reason.

5. When beginning the conversation about life-sustaining treatments, explain why you believe the conversation is needed now by talking about disease progression or the synergistic effect of multiple chronic illnesses. If a geriatric patient is reluctant to begin the conversation, explore the reason for the reluctance.

6. Geriatric patients value independence, preserved function, and preserved cognition. These values may play a significant role in their medical decisions and should be included in advance care planning conversations.

7. Begin the conversation early before a medical crisis occurs and if necessary continue the conversation in future clinical visits.

- POST (Physician Orders for Scope of Treatment)
- SMOST (Summary of Physician Orders for Scope of Treatment)
- TPOPP (Transportable Physician Orders for Patient Preference)
- COLST (Clinician Order for Life Sustaining Treatment)

POLST is not a federal mandate. Each state develops its own forms and regulations; however, the National POLST Paradigm Task Force, established in 2004, has outlined quality standards to follow and assists states in developing POLST programs. The POLST form is completed as a process of informed, shared decision making between physician and patient/representative. During the conversation, the physician and patient explore goals for treatment with special focus on the patient's values and beliefs while exploring the patient's diagnosis, prognosis, and treatment alternatives, including the benefits and risks of life-sustaining treatment. This process allows the physician to order treatments in line with patient goals and to exclude treatments the patient deems extraordinary or burdensome. These orders can then be used in case of medical emergency, whereas the advance directive cannot. In addition, this paradigm recognizes allowing natural death but does not recognize euthanasia/physician-assisted suicide.

Although advance directives are appropriate for all individuals more than 18 years of age, the POLST form should only be used by individuals facing end of life. **Table 1** lists the ways in which the POLST varies from the advance directive. It is notable that the POLST does not replace the advance directive, but that they work together.

Although the POLST form can vary from state to state, most forms include the same principles. The forms include check boxes for life-sustaining treatment (ie, cardiopulmonary resuscitation [CPR], ventilation, artificial hydration/nutrition), medical interventions desired, and whether the patient has an advance directive or medical power of attorney. It should also document who was involved in the discussion to fill out the document and be signed by the attending physician. The medical interventions desired are a choice

	POLST Paradigm Form	Advance Directive Form
Type of Document	Medical orders	Legal document
Who Should Have One?	Seriously ill or frail	All competent adults
Who Fills it Out?	Health care provider, with patient or surrogate	patient only
Does it Identify Proxy?	No	Yes
What Does it State?	Specific medical orders for treatment during a medical emergency	General wishes for treatment as a guide. Used after the medical emergency
Is it Useful to Emergency Medical Services?	Yes	No
When Can it Be Used?	Useful the moment it is signed (ie, current)	Only useful for patients who cannot speak for themselves (ie, future)
How Easy is it to Use?	It is a detailed outline of preferences, and is included in the patient record	Must be interpreted to use; often difficult to locate
Portability	Travels between medical systems, responsibility of physician to make it accessible	Must be carried by patient, is responsibility of the patient only
Are Witnesses Required	No	Yes, or a notary

Table 1
Comparison of the Physician Orders for Life Sustaining Treatment paradigm form and the advance directive form

from (1) comfort measures, (2) limited additional interventions, and (3) full treatment. In addition, a patient may discuss measures that enhance comfort. Comfort measures can include limited trials of noninvasive positive pressure ventilation, transfer to hospital, and stabilization of fractures if the goal is relieving pain and suffering. Patients who desire intravenous (IV) hydration should notate a desire for limited additional interventions because this intervention may prolong life, unless that state has a separate box for fluid/hydration. Other interventions included in this category include noninvasive positive pressure ventilation without time limitation, laboratory tests, imaging, blood products, and cardiac monitoring, but do not include CPR and ventilation. If all life-sustaining treatments are desired, the patient should specify full treatment.

Use of antibiotics is often listed separately on the form. Many patients develop urinary tract infections or aspiration pneumonia as part of the natural death process. It is appropriate to recognize that each infection leads to more debility and increased antibiotic resistance. In this situation, the decision may be made to limit or discontinue antibiotics when the goal is to relieve pain and suffering. The use of hydration and nutrition is also often listed separately from medical interventions on the form and may include limitations (if any) to IV hydration, total parenteral nutrition, and tube feeds.

The POLST paradigm is not legally accepted in all states and the requirements vary from state to state. In Washington DC, Arkansas, Alabama, and South Dakota there is no recognized POLST program (as of February 2017). It is important for each clinician to become familiar with the laws and regulations regarding POLST in the state where they work.

The VA developed a Life-sustaining Treatment Decisions (LTSD) initiative, which will be fully implemented across all VA medical centers by July 2018. The aim of this initiative is to improve patient-centered care for veterans with serious illness, by promoting proactive goals-of-care conversations with patients who are at high risk of a life-threatening clinical event and documenting the goals and treatment decisions in the electronic medical record. This document is durable and will follow the patient throughout the VA system.

Although advance care planning can be a challenging conversation to initiate in the geriatric clinic, the conversation is invaluable. By understanding the components of advance care planning, which include advance directives, do-not-resuscitate orders, and POLST, the clinician can effectively begin the conversation and be reimbursed for the conversation with proper documentation. Taking time to participate in self-study or formal skill training, clinicians can take their communication skills to a new level and achieve a better understanding of each patient's values, which helps to form their health care decisions. Ultimately advance care planning conversations achieve true patient-centered care for geriatric patients.

REFERENCES

1. National Institute of Medicine. Crossing the quality chasm. Washington, DC: National Academy Press; 2001.
2. National Institute of Medicine. Dying in America: improving quality and honoring individual preferences near the end of life. Washington, DC: National Academy Press; 2014.
3. Ward BW, Schiller JS, Goodman RA. Multiple chronic conditions among US adults: a 2012 update. Prev Chronic Dis 2014;11:E62.
4. Teno JM, Grunier A, Schawartz Z, et al. Association between advance directive and quality of end of life care: a national study. J Amer Geriatr Soc 2007;55(2):189–94.
5. H.R. 4449 – Patient self determination act of 1990. Available at: https://www.congress.gov/bill/101st-congress/house-bill/4449. Accessed April 3, 2017.
6. Zhang B, Wright AA, Huskamp HA, et al. Health care cost in the last week of life: associations with end of life conversations. Arch Intern Med 2009;169(5):480–8.
7. Centers for Medicare & Medicaid Services Frequently asked questions about billing the physician fee schedule for advance care planning services. July 14 2016. Available at: https://www.cms.gov/Medicare/Medicare-Fee-for-Service-Payment/PhysicianFeeSched/Downloads/FAQ-Advance-Care-Planning.pdf. Accessed April 3, 2017.
8. Gawande A. Being mortal: medicine and what matters in the end. New York: Metropolitan Books Henry, Holt and company LLC; 2014.
9. Baille WF, Buckman R, Lenzi R, et al. SPIKES – A six step protocol for delivering bad news: application to the patient with cancer. Oncologist 2000;5:302–11.
10. Buckman R. Communication skills. In: Emmanuel LL, Librach SL, editors. Palliative care: core skills and clinical competencies. Philadelphia: Elsevier Saunders; 2011. p. 30–55.
11. US Department of Veterans Affairs. Caring for patients with serious illness: building clinicians' communication skills. In: National Centers for Ethics in Health Care, US Department of Veterans Affairs. 2016. Available at: www.ethics.va.gov/goalsofcaretraining.asp. Accessed April 3, 2017.
12. Starks H, Vig EK, Pearlman RA. Advance care planning. In: Emmanuel LL, Librach SL, editors. Palliative care: core skills and clinical competencies. Philadelphia: Elsevier Saunders; 2011. p. 270–83.
13. National POLST Paradigm POLST paradigm fundamentals. Available at: http://polst.org/about-the-national-polst-paradigm/what-is-polst/. Accessed April 3, 2017.
14. Patients' rights council. POLST: important questions & answers. Available at: http://www.patientsrightscouncil.org/site/polst-important-questions-answers/. Accessed April 3, 2017.

Pain in the Elderly

Identification, Evaluation, and Management of Older Adults with Pain Complaints and Pain-related Symptoms

Andrew Dentino, MD*, Roberto Medina, MD,
Eugene Steinberg, MD

KEYWORDS

- Pain • Elderly • Assessment • Management

KEY POINTS

- Older adults are a special and vulnerable population of patients who warrant the best in a practitioner's clinical toolbox.
- For geriatric patients, this means the lowest threshold for consideration and identification, the most comprehensive and detailed assessment of pain, and an interdisciplinary approach to management.
- When prescribing opioids, practitioners must be extremely vigilant, with continuing surveillance for dosing within the therapeutic windows, for potential adverse side effects (ie, no tolerance to constipation), and for indicators of response, especially in persons who may have cognitive impairment or communicative difficulties.
- Pain management must always occur but only within the explicitly agreed-on goals of care achieved in patient and family meetings regarding these goals of care, and with the patient always as the final arbiter of success.

INTRODUCTION

Pain may be one of the most challenging aspects for many clinicians in the care of older adults.[1] The judicious balance of recognition, comprehensive assessment, focus on function and quality of life, and minimization of exposure to potentially adverse side effects of medications can require much time and effort on the part of health care providers (HCPs) and systems. Attention to special populations within older adults, such as those with cognitive impairment or communication disabilities, or when matters of cultural sensitivity require clinicians to forego certain modalities of treatment (eg, older adults who refuses opioids on religious grounds or for fear of addiction) can be

The Donald W. Reynolds Department of Geriatric Medicine, The University of Oklahoma Health Sciences Center College of Medicine, Oklahoma City, OK, USA
* Corresponding author.
E-mail address: Andrew-Dentino@ouhsc.edu

Prim Care Clin Office Pract 44 (2017) 519–528
http://dx.doi.org/10.1016/j.pop.2017.04.009
0095-4543/17/© 2017 Elsevier Inc. All rights reserved.

challenging, even for the most seasoned HCP. This pragmatic article provides a logical and comprehensive framework for the identification, assessment, and management of pain in older adults, with attention to quality of life and goals of care throughout.

TYPES OF PAIN

Pain may be defined as both an anatomic/physiologic response to an acute stressor (eg, when someone steps on a thorn, which renders an acute pain response in the foot) or as a pathophysiologic constellation of physical and psychological stimuli and learned responses toward potential or putative painful stimuli or experiences.[2]

Pain may be adaptive and salutary when acute, such as in the example of stepping on the thorn. Adaptation is that process whereby the individual may anatomically heal from the acute event (eg, thorn is removed) or develops management strategies to improve function over time (eg, physical therapy after a stroke). Chronic pain is characterized by multiple mechanisms that may be either adaptive or maladaptive. Maladaption ensues when a person is chronically exposed to the pain stimulus, or recovery or rehabilitation cannot occur for any number of reasons.[3] The person then experiences repeated situations in which the stimulus may be avoided, or a prolonged stress response renders a hyperalgesic state (eg, of increased perception or sensation of pain when exposed to the same stimulus). Hyperalgesia has a kindling effect in which interdisciplinary approaches to management may be required to reattune the individual's understanding of pain and adaptation.[4]

Four general pain bases are recognized, either solely or as interacting with other pain types. These bases are the general categories of nociceptive, somatic, neuropathic, and visceral pain. The scope of this article does not allow for a detailed study of the basic science neuromodulatory parameters and the multiplicity and circuitry of brain-body interactions for the different pain types, and readers are encouraged to supplement their knowledge base with a review of basic pain mechanisms.

Nociceptive pain results from stimulation of surface nociceptive pain receptors (nociceptors) such as pacinian corpuscles, which, along with defenses such the gag reflex preventing swallowing after the ingestion of noxious material, are among the body's elemental protection mechanisms for defending against trauma. Nociceptive pain receptors are maximally located in areas of the skin where dexterity and sensation discrimination are paramount, such as in the fingers, toes, and face. They reflexly stimulate limb withdrawal or facial grimace, and lead to secondary brain input to cease the activity resulting in the nociception (eg, withdraw hand from hot stove). Pain is immediate and localizable to the site of injury. Nociception is adaptive and salutary for humans, and alert the individual (and the clinician) to a need for investigation of the basis for nociceptive pain.[5]

Somatic pain is exemplified by a soft tissue or muscle injury. Acute strain or damage results in immediate immobilization (splinting) of the affected limb. Hyperemia and secondary mediators of inflammation ensue, and there is a protective effect of decreased movement leading to restoration and intent for eventual healing. Pain may be intense, throbbing (caused by increased blood flow), or lancing (if neurotendinous structures are involved). For the uncomplicated situation, without secondary or repeated trauma, pretrauma status is ultimately restored.[5]

However, repeated trauma commonly follows after musculoskeletal strain or injury, especially in the elderly. What the single trauma event model does not predict is the neural and musculoskeletal changes of chronic reinjury accompanying somatic pain disorders in older adults, such as in osteoarthritis, vascular disease, or other neurodegenerative conditions. Such secondary maladaptive body responses may have prolonged effects on limb function and strength in older persons.[2]

Neuropathic pain is experience when an afferent or efferent nerve of a motor end plate is directly involved in either posttraumatic or in neurodeteriorative states (such as after stroke or in degenerative neuromuscular conditions), or is caused by primary neurologic insult (eg, trauma or conditions such as neuropathy). Nerve pain may be described as shooting, and lancinating pain syndromes may be caused by identifiable (eg, via electromyography) or unidentifiable (eg, phantom pain after limb loss) causes. Neuropathic pain may coexist with other types of pain and may contribute to or exacerbate other pain causes.[2]

Visceral pain results from physical stretching of organ surfaces (such as the gall bladder, hepatic capsule, or the pleural surfaces) or from decreased blood flow (such as in atherosclerotic disease). In these cases, pain may be intermittent, colicky, or diffuse and poorly localizable (especially when involving the abdominal viscera). Visceral pain may be enigmatic and difficult to assess, especially in older adults with cognitive impairment or with communication disorders.

PRESENTATION OF PAIN IN OLDER ADULTS

Multiple bases for not only the differences in presentation of pain in older versus younger persons exist but also for the heterogeneity of pain symptom–related and syndrome-related presentations across older adults. Similar to the differences in other sickness behaviors in young versus old,[4] the reasons for differing pain manifestations in the elderly refer to all organ systems and to the whole person as well. Decreased levels of neurotransmitters, decreased motor end plate function, and decreased cerebral and peripheral arterial blood flow all contribute to differing perceptions of and responses to pain in elders. Differing thresholds for reporting pain in older adults, and even a potential stigma for reporting (potential loss of independence, potential new diagnosis of a life-limiting condition, potential reporting biases in older cohorts, and so forth) may furthermore warrant clinicians to have greater sensitivity to investigation of possible pain symptom equivalents in older adults compared with their younger counterparts.[4]

Older persons may firstly have more nonspecific symptoms or complaints, or might not report at all (but only affirm they have pain to the clinicians' inquiry). They may have limited cognitive reserve to be able to characterize their sensations as pain, or may have an inability to verbalize their complaints. HCPs must ask, and ask again, about experiences (eg, a fall), situations (eg, climbing stairs or rising from a toilet), or activities (eg, bending or grabbing/fist making) that create specific symptoms, because older persons might not voluntarily disclose this information.[6]

Furthermore, disease states may variably change the way pain is perceived by older adults. Cardiac disease with decreased peripheral perfusion, neuropathies decreasing the ability to sense pain, or arthritic joints (with secondary conditions such as crystal deposition, infection, or occult fracture) all may contribute or even additively or synergistically obfuscate the diagnostic entity (eg, myocardial infarction, cholecystitis, urinary tract infection) causing the pain.[7]

APPROACH TO OLDER PATIENTS WITH PAIN COMPLAINTS

Perhaps the most important determinant of successful identification of pain cause in older adults derives from communication with the elder. Older persons may be less likely to identify specific antecedents, concomitant symptoms, or even the pain or its severity or potential seriousness. Therefore, a relaxed, slow, and careful approach to communication with the older adult as to the pain symptoms, and a purposefully repetitive nature of inquiry as to history and current functioning, may be met with the greatest likelihood of elucidation of the true nature of the processes involved in the older person's pain complaints.

A sequential but broad approach to history and physical examination is required: biological causes, psychological manifestation, social consequences, and even spiritual belief systems come into play in older adults' depictions of their pain status. A careful assessment of medical bases for pain; the meaning of pain in the older adult's view of health and illness; psychological factors such as anxiety, depression, and cognitive impairment overlaid onto the physical symptoms' descriptions; and the potential social effects (removal from independent living, concern for revocation of driving license and personal independence; caregiver needs, and so forth) all come into play in the assessment of older adults with pain. Even matters of religious or spiritual belief systems may cause patients to see pain as a weakness or shortcoming. A nonjudgmental, friendly, and cautious approach to older patients, with multiple reiterations of what the patient is saying to not only verify and corroborate but also to establish therapeutic alliance, is well worth the time of investment in older persons with pain issues.[6] Evaluation should also always include a history of past usage of analgesics, psychotropic medications, and alcohol and drugs, because this history influences the formulation of, and the communication with the patient about, a therapeutic regimen that may include controlled substances and the attendant shared decision making, informed consent, and the legal and ethical responsibilities of the treatment contract.

The physical examination must be the classic head-to-toe assessment of the elder. Cultural or cohort factors may render older persons reticent about disclosing aspects of their personal self-care, but these are revealed through a respectful physical examination that includes complete skin examination and genitourinary assessment. Older adults may not be forthcoming with pain issues when they involve personal body functions, and clinicians best placed to elucidate these physical findings.

Laboratory and ancillary studies should loosely follow the history and physical examination findings. If metabolic, endocrine, infectious, or musculoskeletal issues are posited in the diagnostic differential, a selected analysis of laboratory work and radiologic investigations is the best means to prudently identify potential bases but should avoid the indiscriminate use of all tests possible in the absence of relevant signs or symptoms. Musculoskeletal examination findings should dictate the appropriate use of radiograph studies, and function should always be the determinant for ordering any test or study (ie, is the test or radiology study going to affect the management of the patient?).[8]

MANAGEMENT OF PAIN IN OLDER ADULTS

The mainstay of management of pain conditions in older adults must always be to strive for consideration of all nonpharmacologic therapies (physical, occupational, speech) in which the older adult may be able to participate.[8] In addition, all older adults who have undergone therapies should be reevaluated at regular intervals to assess whether a reinitiation of the completed therapy would be advantageous for preservation of function or for potential improvement, but also whether it is warranted for maintenance of quality of life. Therapies and physical medicine modalities are cost-effective when chosen judiciously and with attainable restorative or rehabilitation goals.[3] Therapies may also lessen the burden of medications (pharmacotherapy for chronic pain conditions), given the increased probability for adverse side effects of analgesics in older adults.[9]

However, many older adults report increased satisfaction with pain management regimens when medications (pharmacotherapy) are considered when nonpharmacologic therapies alone have not resulted in sufficient diminution of pain level or sufficient improvement in function. Medications and therapies are never an either/or option, but are always a both/and option when used complementarily and when the treatment team and its strategies reflect an optimism for maintenance and potential for improvement in pain control and function.

Most paradigms for pain medicine involve an escalation of the class of medicines, usually only in a ladder fashion, considering a stronger class of medication only when a less potent class has either proved ineffective or the decrease in pain symptoms results in the patient accepting the potential side effect risk and burdens of the stronger class of agents.

The first agent to be considered (unless contraindicated) is acetaminophen. Starting an older adult, especially one who may have cognitive or communication difficulties, on low-dose acetaminophen is often met with increased physical activity or even subjective improvements in eating or sleep (because the person is now at a lessened pain level that makes it possible to attend to activities of daily living [ADLs]). Acetaminophen may be useful in nociceptive, somatic, or visceral pain types. Acetaminophen should be considered at an initial starting dose of 325 mg or 500 mg, and increased up to a total dose of 2000 mg/d. Care is needed in patients with hepatic insufficiency. Accidental overdose is possible if significant amounts are ingested; hospitalization is recommended and support care initiated if nomogram levels indicate toxicity.[10]

Occasionally persons are not fully satisfied with their level of long-term pain control with acetaminophen alone. In these cases, always review the need for potential physical and/or occupational therapy evaluation, and always recommend group exercise when appropriate. Socialization, diet, and sleep hygiene all have roles in the long-term management of older adults with pain, in terms of overall functional status.

Nonsteroidal antiinflammatory drugs (NSAIDs) may be considered for specific pain types (eg, somatic, after a musculoskeletal injury); however, given their overall adverse side effect profile (cardiac, cerebrovascular, gastrointestinal), in older adults their use should be directed, time limited, at the lowest dose possible, and with medical supervision of care. Ibuprofen or its equivalent at a dose not to exceed 600 to 800 mg/d maximum at any given time, and a ceiling of 2400 mg/d, should be assiduously adhered to, with a stop date agreed on a priori to review the amount of analgesia the NSAID has added. Acetaminophen and NSAIDs may be cautiously used in the same patient but not simultaneously coadministered. At any sign of bleeding (especially in any patient on antiplatelet or anticoagulant therapy, in which case even initiating NSAID therapy should have its risks/benefits weighed and only then be agreed on beforehand) or if any new symptoms develop, the NSAIDs use should perfunctorily be evaluated as a potential contributor, and appropriate immediate medical management effected.[8]

It may be that an adherent, compliant, and informed patient does not experience an adequate level of pain amelioration, even with acetaminophen, therapies/exercise, an NSAID trial, and salutary lifestyle changes (offloading the affected joint if musculoskeletal, and so forth). In such patients, especially for those in whom a longer than short-term (ie, hospice care level) prognosis exists, a serious discussion of the pros and cons of opioid therapy should occur. Only with true informed consent on the part of a competent patient, or with the consent of the legal next of kin/power of attorney if the patient is not decisional, should the HCP embark on a trial of opioid therapy, with the understanding that this class of analgesia may be considered indefinitely, with close medical monitoring and follow-up, and deescalated/titrated down to discontinuation if goals of care are not met or if supervening adverse events preclude adherence or patient safety.

All opioid agents work on the same receptor type (mu), found in the central nervous system but also throughout the body (and therefore there is the risk of side effects in multiple organ systems). All opioid prescribing must be by the practitioner first, always with the requisite training and competence in the medical decision making involved in opioid therapy. There should always be 1 drug, 1 prescriber, 1 pharmacy as a goal for long-term, medically stable patients once acute pain needs and goals are achieved.[11]

All opioid prescribing should reflect the equianalgesic equivalency of that agent and dose back to the standard of morphine sulfate. Extracted from the poppy plant, morphine is a natural opiate medication that is commonly used for acute and chronic pain in combination with nonpharmacologic modalities. It is the standard opiate to equilibrate dosing among the different types of natural, semisynthetic, and synthetic formulations. Its manufacture, importation, and distribution are regulated, as are other controlled substances according to the federally defined Comprehensive Drug Abuse Prevention and Controlled Substance Act of 1970. The Drug Enforcement Agency (in the Department of Justice) as well as local state narcotic prescribing authorities have classified controlled substances in 5 categories (schedules I–V) based on addiction or abuse potential, therapeutic use, and overall safety, with the public's interest primarily in mind; higher scheduling indicating less overall addiction potential. Morphine is classified as a schedule II medication and thus has been noted to have high potential for abuse that can lead to physical or psychological dependence if used inappropriately (other schedule II drugs: oxycodone, hydromorphone, methadone, meperidine, fentanyl, opium, codeine, and hydrocodone). Prescribers must follow all regulations and restrictions to use in the jurisdiction and health system in which morphine is prescribed. It is requisite that all HCPs be fully trained and competent in their scope of practice for the prescription of controlled substances.[11]

Morphine is approximately 3 times more potent in its intravenous form than in its oral form. That is, approximately 10 mg of intravenous morphine are equivalent to 30 mg of oral morphine. All other opioids are thus compared with oral morphine to determine their equianalgesic dose. Morphine intravenously has an effect in approximately 10 minutes, and orally in approximately 20 minutes. Its duration of action (analgesia) is approximately 4 to 6 hours. However, its half-life may be prolonged in several states, including renal insufficiency. Metabolites with much longer half-lives are produced after hepatic metabolism, and these may accumulate and be associated with or responsible for certain side effects, including neurotoxicity, which may manifest as tremor, myoclonus, confusion, stupor, or coma.[4]

Morphine should be begun at low doses (10 mg oral equivalents) and increased by approximately 50% per day or 2 days over the first days of therapy, always under medical monitoring and supervision, until steady state ensues. Intravenous morphine must be closely monitored at the initiation of therapy, because of its rapid ability to incite adverse side effects (respiratory depression being the most dangerous) with too rapid dosage titration. Other main side effects to be anticipated from morphine and all opioids, in addition to respiratory depression, include sedation and constipation. Urinary retention and several other side effects are common and prescribers must be vigilant with surveillance for the development of potential opioid-related side effects. Patients may slowly habituate to the respiratory depressive and sedative side effects of opioids, but constipation must always be aggressively prevented and as aggressively treated if it occurs. Naloxone should always be immediately available in the setting of opioid therapy to provide a potentially lifesaving rescue antidote if overdose is ever suspected. Naloxone must always be used with medical monitoring capabilities.[12]

As-needed doses of morphine should be allowed, to get the patient as safely and as quickly as possible to a comfortable level of analgesia (eg, within several days). As-needed doses of morphine should not exceed 50% of the total daily dose; the total daily dose can then be recalculated by assessing the total analgesic amount needed (both regularly scheduled and as needed), and a new baseline routine dose can be established. As low a total daily dose as possible so as to provide the patient with a reasonable level of pain control, but still allow the patient to be able to attend to their ADLs, not experience excessive sedation, and so forth, is the goal. Total analgesia is neither pragmatically attainable nor the ultimate desired goal; an acceptable level of analgesia that allows the person to function comfortably is the realistic goal, and this must be communicated and agreed on by prescriber and patient/family beforehand.[13]

Once a steady state has been achieved, long-acting (usually twice daily) morphine preparations should replace the initial, short-acting morphine on which the patient was originally begun (long-acting morphine generally should not be used as initial therapy, especially in opioid-naive patients). As always, because older adults may behave and respond more heterogeneously than younger patients, caution and prudent initial opioid prescribing and monitoring is always required.

Most older patients require less than 90 mg/d of long-acting oral morphine if their underlying disease is stable. Older adults requiring larger doses early in opioid therapy should prompt the prescriber to reevaluating for any secondary bases for medical nonresponse or submaximal response.

The other commonly prescribed opioids, oxycodone, hydrocodone, and hydromorphone, may be cautiously compared with morphine as follows: 30 mg of oral morphine (or 10 mg of intravenous morphine) is equianalgesic to:

30 mg of oral hydrocodone
20 mg of oral oxycodone
7.5 mg of oral hydromorphone
1.5 mg of intravenous hydromorphone[14]

It is important for prescribers to be able to create accurate equianalgesic doses of all of these agents. It is important to become familiar with all 4 agents because the opioids exist in several different chemical classes, and intolerance (intolerable side effects) to one class might develop, whereas another class might not be met with a similar degree of side effects. Furthermore, in some cases, opioid rotation may benefit the patient when, after a period of time, the patient may respond better on a different class of opioid; for example, when the dose of one opioid has been increased repeatedly without the anticipated therapeutic response that such an upward titration should produce. Prescribers are strongly recommended to consult a pain medicine specialist or pharmacist who is well versed in analgesic pharmacy if opioid rotation is to be considered.[2,13,15]

Despite initiating therapy with hydrocodone, oxycodone, or hydromorphone, clinicians may still prescribe as-needed medications. Always consider cross-tolerance among the different opioids, and decrease the as-needed calculation by approximately 50% to account for this. The as-needed doses may be increased (to render a new baseline routine daily dosage) or decreased (as analgesic needs are met).[3]

There is no ceiling dose for opioids. With care, titration, and meticulous attention to surveillance for possible side effects and their prevention, even patients with advanced disease burden can safely be managed on higher doses of analgesia. Usually, more than 90 mg/d morphine equivalent is considered a high dosage.[16]

Another agent that may be considered is transdermal fentanyl. This opioid is dosed in micrograms per hour as opposed to milligrams, and as a patch, and is usually administered (ie, the patch is changed) every 72 hours. In general, the dose in micrograms per hour of transdermal fentanyl (usually administered every 72 hours) is approximately half the total daily dose of oral morphine equivalent. For instance, a patient who is stable on 50 mg/d of oral morphine could cautiously be converted to 12 µg/h with a fentanyl patch (changed every 72 hours), because this allows for 50% cross-tolerance, with the patient also to receive as-needed doses of short-acting morphine to total half the daily dose (eg, 19 mg of morphine as needed every 8 hours). However, interindividual variability of metabolism is significant and, as discussed earlier, a pain medicine specialist or pharmacist who is well versed in analgesic pharmacy should be consulted if there are any questions or concerns as to fentanyl. Also, fentanyl transdermal patches may be relatively contraindicated in frail elders with limited adipose stores, because the absorption of the patch depends on there being sufficient absorptive body surface.[4,15]

One other opioid that warrants mention is methadone. This synthetic opioid possesses unique and variable pharmacokinetic and pharmacodynamic properties, and should only be prescribed under the supervision of a pain medicine specialist or pharmacist who is well versed in analgesic pharmacy. Although there may be cases in which methadone achieves analgesia in patients who are refractory to or intolerant of other opioids, the requisite detailed discussion of this unique and special medicine is beyond the scope of this article.[3,4,8,17]

Opioid doses should be titrated up carefully and slowly, and deescalation (weaning) and eventual discontinuation should always occur whenever it can safely be achieved over a period of time. Abrupt opioid discontinuation (withdrawal) can be a distressing and potentially medically dangerous event. Only under the closest of medical (ie, inpatient hospital) monitoring should opioids ever be abruptly discontinued in an older adult, and only if the life of the patient requires it.[6,18]

One concern that HCPs may have regarding opioids is addiction. Close screening for a history of substance abuse earlier in life, clear and detailed discussions (always with an informed consent/written contract) as to the anticipated therapy, the intended degrees of response, and actions to be undertaken if intolerance or lack of desired therapeutic effect occurs, should minimize the risk of medical addiction. Pseudoaddiction is a state in which a patient displays behaviors toward obtaining the agent in question, but when prescribed is adherent, taking it appropriately and without otherwise addictive behaviors. Pseudoaddiction is the patient's behavioral communication of the need for a prescribed agent that is now lacking. These patients should be restored to the informed consent/written contract of the opioid prescriber, with ongoing and continued surveillance for true addictive behaviors.[19]

In addition to opioids, other adjunctive analgesics exist that may also be considered with consultation of a pain medicine specialist or pharmacist who is well versed in analgesic pharmacy. For instance, neuropathic pain may respond well to duloxetine or other neurolytic or anticonvulsant agents. Other agents may also be explored (eg, ketamine) within the purview of the subspecialty of pain medicine. Similarly, even patients in palliative care may benefit from judicious procedural approaches to intractable pain (eg, nerve blocks). These approaches should not be withheld from older adult patients whose pain is otherwise uncontrolled.[20]

SUMMARY

To relieve pain is to engage in the most time-honored and noble of pursuits for HCPs. Older adults are a special and vulnerable population of patients who warrant the best in a practitioner's clinical toolbox. For geriatric patients, this means the lowest threshold for consideration and identification, the most comprehensive and detailed assessment of pain, and an interdisciplinary approach to management. When prescribing opioids, practitioners must be extremely vigilant, with continuing surveillance for dosing within the therapeutic windows, for potential adverse side effects (ie, no tolerance to constipation), and for indicators of response, especially in persons who may have cognitive impairment or communicative difficulties. Pain management must always occur but only within the explicitly agreed-on goals of care achieved in patient and family meetings regarding these goals of care, and with the patient always as the final arbiter of success. Pain management in older adults is an extraordinarily fulfilling professional undertaking, to improve the lives of society's fastest-growing segment.

REFERENCES

1. Ghosh A, Dzeng E, Cheng MJ. Interaction of palliative care and primary care. Clin Geriatr Med 2015;31:207–18.
2. Woolf CJ. Pain. Neurobiol Dis 2000;7:504–10.
3. Rastogi R, Meek BD. Management of chronic pain in elderly frail patients finding a suitable personalized method of control. Clin Interv Aging 2013;8:37–46.
4. Huang AR, Mallet L. Prescribing opioids in older people. Maturitas 2013;71: 123–9.
5. Frias B, Merighi A. Capsaicin, nociception and pain. Molecules 2016;21:797.
6. Mossello E, Ballini E. Management of patients with Alzheimer's disease: pharmacological treatment and quality of life. Ther Adv Chronic Dis 2012;3(4):183–93.
7. McKeown JL. Pain management issues. Anesthesiol Clin 2015;33:563–76.
8. Abdulla A, Adams N, Bone M, et al. Guidance on the management of pain in older people. Age Ageing 2013;42:i1–57.
9. Baumbauer KM, Young EE, Starkweather AR, et al. Managing chronic pain in special populations with emphasis on pediatric geriatric and drug abuser populations. Med Clin North Am 2016;100:183–97.
10. Yoon E, Babar A, Choudhary M, et al. Acetaminophen-induced hepatotoxicity: a comprehensive update. J Clin Transl Hepatol 2016;4:131–42.
11. Meara E, Horwitz JR, Powell W, et al. State legal restrictions and prescription opioid use among disabled adults. N Engl J Med 2016;375:44–53.
12. Ciejka M, Nguyen K, Bluth MH, et al. Drug toxicities of common analgesic medications in the emergency department. Clin Lab Med 2016;36:761–76.
13. Webster, LR. Breakthrough pain in the management of chronic persistent pain syndromes. 2008. Available at: https://www.ajmc.com. Accessed April 4, 2016.
14. Shaheen PE, Walsh D, Lasheen W, et al. Opioid equianalgesic tables: are they all equally dangerous? J Pain Symptom Manage 2009;38(3):409–17.
15. Koncicki HM, Unruh M, Schell JO. Pain management in CKD: a guide for nephrology providers. Am J Kidney Dis 2016;69(3):451–60.
16. Hwang U, Platts-Mills TF. Acute pain management in older adults in the emergency department. Clin Geriatr Med 2013;29:151–64.
17. Knotkova H, Fine PG, Portenoy RK. Opioid rotation: the science and the limitations of equianalgesic table use. J Pain Symptom Manage 2009;38(3):426–39.

18. Baker N. Using cognitive behavior therapy and mindfulness techniques in the management of chronic pain in primary care. Prim Care 2016;43:203–16.
19. Greene MS, Chambers RA. Pseudoaddiction: fact or fiction? An investigation of the medical literature. Curr Addict Rep 2015;2:310–7.
20. Guy S, Mehta S, Leff L, et al. Anticonvulsant medication use for the management of pain following spinal cord injury systematic review and effectiveness analysis. Spinal Cord 2014;52:89–96.

Hypertension in the Older Adult

Belinda Setters, MD, MS[a,b], Holly M. Holmes, MD, MS[c,*]

KEYWORDS

- Hypertension • Elderly hypertension • Blood pressure • Geriatric

KEY POINTS

- Hypertension is common among elderly patients, and with projected population, aging is anticipated to be an ever-increasing public health problem.
- Hypertension is associated with significant cardiovascular risk for heart attack, stroke, and chronic kidney disease and remains the most common reason adults to see their primary care provider aside from routine medication refill visits.
- Confusion still exists regarding treatment of elders, specifically who to treat and how low to push blood pressures.
- Quality of life, adverse treatment effects, and goals of care should be central to the treatment of hypertension in older and frail adults.

INTRODUCTION

Approximately 1 in 3 adults have hypertension (HTN) with another 8% estimated to be undiagnosed, making it the most common reason after medication refills for adult primary care visits.[1] Currently, 76.4 million adults have HTN in the United States alone.[2] This statistic, combined with HTN's association with aging physiology and the aging of the populous, makes HTN one of the most pressing current public health concerns.[3,4]

HTN is defined as isolated systolic elevation, isolated diastolic elevation, or both.[5] Although ongoing research has provided large-scale data on both the measurement and treatment of HTN, practitioners have been left with the difficult task of assessing conflicting reports about who to treat, how low to drive pressures, and how to balance the increasing concern of overtreatment. This is especially problematic in the

The authors have nothing to disclose.
[a] Department of Internal Medicine, Robley Rex VAMC, University of Louisville School of Medicine, 800 Zorn Avenue, 6 West – GEC #627, Louisville, KY 40206, USA; [b] Inpatient Geriatrics, Department of Family & Geriatric Medicine, Robley Rex VAMC, University of Louisville School of Medicine, 800 Zorn Avenue, 6 West – GEC #627, Louisville, KY 40206, USA; [c] Geriatric & Palliative Medicine, Department of Internal Medicine, University of Texas Houston McGovern Medical School, 6431 Fannin, MBS 5.111, Houston, TX 77030, USA
* Corresponding author.
E-mail address: Holly.M.Holmes@uth.tmc.edu

Prim Care Clin Office Pract 44 (2017) 529–539
http://dx.doi.org/10.1016/j.pop.2017.05.002
0095-4543/17/© 2017 Elsevier Inc. All rights reserved.

treatment of older and more frail adults for whom adverse side effects and poor outcomes are more worrisome.

HYPERTENSION DEFINED AND MEASURED

HTN has traditionally been defined as systolic blood pressure (SBP) ≥140 mm Hg or diastolic blood pressure (DBP) ≥90 mm Hg taken as the average of 3 properly measured readings on 2 or more outpatient office visits.[6–8] Although the basic tenants of this definition continue to stand today, additional research into the best methods for screening for HTN and the most appropriate numerical definitions has given rise to some confusion about how to define this common cardiovascular disease.

Blood pressure measurements in the outpatient office setting can miss elevations occurring at other times or incorrectly diagnose white coat HTN as primary essential HTN. More recent recommendations therefore are to use home ambulatory blood pressure monitoring as the preferred measurement for diagnosis. These ambulatory home measurements more closely correlate with daytime blood pressure readings and are more accurate.

Ambulatory readings averaging ≥130/80 over a 24-hour period are diagnostic of HTN. If measuring daytime pressures only, HTN would be defined by greater than 135/85, whereas nocturnal measures of 120/70 would constitute HTN diagnosis owing to decreased pressures during nighttime sleep rhythms. If it is not possible to monitor patients at home in this manner, traditional one-point-in-time measures would be acceptable. By this traditional method, HTN could be defined as ≥140/90 as noted above.

Appropriate measurement of blood pressures is important because HTN disease is associated with significant morbidity and mortality, including heart attack, stroke, chronic kidney disease (CKD), and death. Accordingly, HTN remains the most important risk factor for many of these associated cardiovascular disorders. Effective treatment to reduce blood pressure to goal is the single most important modifiable intervention to improve both the length and quality of life for adults, especially older adults, who are disproportionately affected.

Pathology

HTN results from the body's response to external stressors to maintain the blood pressure at effective ranges for perfusion of vital organs such as the brain and heart. When plasma volume or cardiac output are ineffective, common regulating pathways such as the Renin-angiotensin system and autonomic nervous system respond accordingly to increase blood pressure. Cardiac output volume and systemic vascular resistance result in measurable blood pressure ($CO \times SVR = BP$). If the body cannot maintain perfusion to organs as needed at normal blood pressures, it will compensate by either increasing output volume or resistance, thereby increasing pressures.[5]

As changes occur in body position, baroreceptor-medicated responses in the autonomic nervous system increase tone in veins and arteries while lower-extremity and abdominal muscular contractions increase blood return from the lower extremities. These instantaneous, automatic responses maintain blood pressure and therefore adequate cerebral perfusion with position changes.[9] If these mechanisms do not work correctly or work inefficiently, an acute decrease in blood pressure can occur. A decrease of ≥20 mm Hg in systolic or ≥10 mm Hg diastolic pressures occurring with changes in position is defined as orthostatic hypotension.[10]

Orthostatic hypotension is more common among elderly and frail patients, occurring in up to 40% of elderly patients with cardiovascular risk factors.[11,12] Normal aging changes combined with medication side effects and multimorbidity make elders with cardiovascular risk factors more likely to have orthostatic hypotension. Practitioners should use caution in treating HTN while watching for orthostasis, as hypoperfusion not only causes significant morbidity in dizziness, falls, and syncope but has been implemented in long-term cognitive impairment such as dementia and stroke.[13–15]

Vascular resistance increases with age as the vascular wall becomes less compliant. This change, combined with common age-associated conditions such as heart failure which reduce cardiac output, results in the increased incidence of HTN among elders. Although a more detailed discussion of the pathology of HTN is beyond the scope of this review, it should be noted that these recommendations generally apply to both primary (formerly known as essential HTN) and secondary HTN (resulting from the effects of medications or other diseases).

The elderly and frail are more likely to have medication side effects and age-associated diseases such as CKD (**Table 1**). Therefore, ruling out secondary causes such as nonsteroidal anti-inflammatory drug or steroid effects and common age-associated diseases such as obstructive sleep apnea and CKD is important in assessing older patients presenting with HTN. Appropriately distinguishing primary HTN from secondary causes not only avoids unnecessary prescribing and the polypharmacy cascade that follows but improves reduction to goal, treatment adherence, and long-term outcomes.

Screening

Because there are few risks of blood pressure measurement, most experts recommend screening all adults older than 18 years at least once for HTN. Patients 18 to 39 years with normal blood pressure readings and no risk factors for HTN only need to be screened every 3 years. Patients older than 40 years should be screened annually.

Table 1
Common factors associated with and causes of hypertension by type

Primary HTN	Secondary HTN
Primary disease resulting from genetic & environmental effect	*Results from underlying effects of other disease*
Common factors related to primary HTN	Common causes of secondary HTN
• Age	• Primary renal disease
• Obesity	• Primary hyperaldosteronism
• Race (black)	• Pheochromocytoma
• Genetics/family history	• Obstructive sleep apnea
• Reduced nephron number	• Cushing's disease
• Physical inactivity	• Coarctation of the aorta
• High sodium and/or alcohol intake	• Prescription or over-thecounter medications
• Personality type/traits (type A)	○ Nonsteroidal anti-inflammatory drugs
• Cardiovascular risks (diabetes, hyperlipidemia)	○ Decongestants
	○ Erythropoietin
	○ Glucocorticoids
	○ Cyclosporine
	○ Stimulants (amphetamines)
	○ Antidepressants (Tricyclic and Serotonin Reuptake Inhibitors)

Regardless of age, patients with risks such as stressful lifestyle (type A personality), excessive alcohol intake, high sodium diet, diabetes, or obesity should be screened more frequently at their provider's discretion. Most providers choose to take blood pressure readings for these patients at each office visit. Recommendations are shown in **Table 2**.

TREATMENT

Treatment of HTN to reduce blood pressure has consistently been shown to reduce cardiovascular morbidity and mortality.[6,16] Multiple studies have been conducted in older persons to determine the optimal level at which to initiate treatment and the ideal blood pressure goals. There remains some disagreement regarding current recommendations for initiation and maintenance treatment. Furthermore, the minimal blood pressure, or lower threshold below which blood pressure should not be lowered, has not been adequately determined.

The blood pressure at which lifestyle changes or pharmacologic therapy should be initiated has evolved and been updated as more data from randomized controlled trials accumulates to support specific blood pressure goals. Lifestyle modifications are recommended in adults with lower blood pressure levels, with SBP 120 to 139 or DBP 80 to 89 mm Hg. Recommendations include dietary sodium reduction, reducing alcohol consumption, aerobic exercise, weight loss or maintenance of a healthy weight, smoking cessation, and stress reduction. Lower sodium diets have been associated with decreased cardiovascular events in several studies.[17] The effect that lowered sodium has on blood pressure may be of greater magnitude in older rather than younger adults.[6] In addition, adequate potassium, calcium, and magnesium intake are recommended, although they should not be used in place of treatment when pharmacologic treatment is appropriate. Finally, reducing or avoiding medications that can increase blood pressure—such as nonsteroidal anti-inflammatory drugs, corticosteroids, some antirheumatic drugs, and sympathomimetic drugs—are other interventions that can be taken when possible.[6,17]

Table 3 shows selected hypertension treatment guidelines from professional societies. The Joint National Commission (JNC-8) recommends a general approach to initiate antihypertensive therapy in patients 60 years and older when SBP is ≥150 mm Hg or DBP is ≥90 mmg Hg, with a goal of SBP less than 150 and DBP less than 90, which were grade A recommendations. If a lower BP is achieved and a patient is tolerating medication without side effects or a decrement in quality of life, the recommendation is to continue therapy without adjustment, which was a grade E recommendation based on expert consensus. In all adults with CKD or with diabetes, initiation should occur at SBP ≥140 mm Hg or DBP ≥90 to treat to a goal of SBP less than 140 and DBP less than 90, both of which were grade E

Table 2 Screening recommendations for adults	
Age, y	**Screening Recommendation**
18	One-time screen
18–39	Every 3 y If risk factors such as obesity, diabetes, or high alcohol intake, more frequent screening is recommended at provider's discretion.
>40	Annually
>80	Annually or at provider discretion

Table 3
Selected professional society guidelines with specific recommendations for the treatment of hypertension in older adults

Guideline	When to Initiate Therapy	Goal	Preferred Medications
JNC-8[8]	SBP ≥150 mm Hg OR DBP ≥90 mm Hg	SBP <150 mm Hg and DBP <90 mm Hg	Thiazide, CCB, or ACEI/ARB Blacks without CKD: thiazide or CCB CKD: ACEI or ARB
NICE[18]	Any patient with BP ≥160/100 mm Hg and avg home measure of ≥150/95 mm Hg Age <80 and organ damage, CVD, CKD, DM, or 10 y risk ≥20%: BP ≥140/90 mm Hg or home avg ≥135/85 mm Hg	BP <140/90 mm Hg in people <80 y BP <150/90 mm Hg in people ≥80 y	CCB, then ACE/ARB, then thiazide
ACCF/AHA[6]	SBP ≥140 or DBP ≥90	<140/90 mm Hg if uncomplicated HTN <120/80 mm Hg if LV dysfunction <130/80 mm Hg if DM, CAD, CKD, PAD Avoid SBP <135 mm Hg or DBP <65 mm Hg in those 80 and older SBP 140–145 mm Hg is acceptable in those 80+ y	Thiazides first line, also CCBs and ACEI/ARBs BB if CAD or CHF
ESH/ESC[19]	SBP ≥140 mm Hg for younger SBP ≥160 mm Hg if ≥80 y	SBP between 150 and 140 mm Hg, and <140 mm Hg in fit older people If ≥80 y, between 150 and 140 mm Hg if in good physical and mental condition DBP <90, or <85 mm Hg if DM is present	Diuretics, BB, CCBs, ACEIs, ARBs as monotherapy or combination therapy (in the absence of compelling indications) Thiazides and CCBs preferred in the elderly with isolated systolic hypertension

Abbreviations: BB, beta blocker; CAD, coronary artery disease; CCB, calcium channel blocker; CHF, congestive heart failure; DM, diabetes mellitus; ESH, European Society of Hypertension; ESC, European Society of Cardiology; PAD, peripheral arterial disease.
Data from Refs.[6,8,18,19]

recommendations. Although preferred initial therapy could include a thiazide, calcium channel blocker, angiotensin-converting enzyme inhibitor (ACEI), or angiotensin receptor blocker (ARB), patients with CKD should receive an ACEI or ARB. Black patients without CKD, even patients with diabetes, should initiate treatment with a thiazide or calcium channel blocker.[8]

Guidelines from the National Institute for Health and Care Excellence (NICE) in the United Kingdom's National Health Service specify recommendations based on age. In patients younger than 80, the recommendation is to initiate medication when patients have a blood pressure ≥140/90 mm Hg and ambulatory daytime average or home monitoring blood pressure of ≥135/85 along with end organ damage, cardiovascular disease, CKD, diabetes mellitus, or a 10-year cardiovascular risk ≥20%. Any patient with clinic blood pressure ≥160/100 mm Hg and average ambulatory monitoring or home measuring of ≥150/95 should receive medication. Patients 55 and older or of African or Caribbean descent should initiate therapy with a calcium channel blocker first, after which an ACEI or ARB could be added, followed by a thiazide diuretic.[18]

Treatment Targets in Older Patients

Despite the high prevalence of hypertension in patients 75 and older and particularly 80 and older, there are relatively few treatment trials that focus on patients of advanced age to determine optimal blood pressure targets, optimal levels at which treatment should be initiated, and optimal medication therapy regimens.[20] A 2009 Cochrane review evaluated treatment trials for hypertension in people 60 and older, including 15 trials.[16] Trials in the review and meta-analysis included the Systolic Hypertension in the Elderly Program (SHEP) and the Hypertension in the Very Elderly Trial (HYVET). The conclusion was that there was significant benefit in treating moderate-to-severe systolic or diastolic hypertension in adults older than 60 years in reducing cardiovascular and cerebrovascular morbidity and mortality. The benefit in terms of all-cause mortality was only seen in adults 60 to 80 years and was not seen in adults 80 and older. The number needed to treat for cerebrovascular morbidity and mortality was 50 people, over a 4.5-year period, and the number needed to treat for cardiovascular morbidity and mortality was 100. Most of the trials used step therapy to achieve a BP goal, with a thiazide diuretic being the first-line choice for most trials.

The American College of Cardiology Foundation (ACCF)/American Heart association (AHA) Guideline developed by expert consensus was an update that intended to put the results of the HYVET trial into perspective into updated guidelines. Notably, the target blood pressure in HYVET was SBP less than 150 or DBP less than 80.[16] Although the ACCF/AHA consensus recommendation was that there are benefits of treating adults older than 80 years to lower BP targets, the conclusion was that it was unclear whether the goal SBP should be the same for people 65 to 79 years versus 80 years and older.[6]

Most recently, blood pressure targets in older people have been put into question again by the results of the Systolic Blood Pressure Intervention Trial (SPRINT) trial. In SPRINT, adults were randomly assigned to intensive (systolic <120 mm Hg) versus standard (systolic <140 mm Hg) blood pressure goals.[21] In a separate analysis of the participants 75 years and older, the more intensive group had significantly reduced cardiovascular morbidity and mortality.[22] Adverse events were higher but not statistically significantly different in the intensive treatment group, including hypotension, syncope, acute kidney injury, and electrolyte abnormalities. Despite the fact that patients with diabetes mellitus or with recent stroke had been excluded from the study, based on data from the National Health and Nutrition Examination Survey, 7.6% of the

US adult population would meet eligibility criteria for the SPRINT study, with eligibility increasing with older age. This finding represents 8.6 million people with hypertension not being treated currently.[23]

Optimal targets and levels of control of hypertension in older people remain uncertain. Reflecting this lack of certainty, several international treatment guidelines in the United States, Canada, Australia, Europe, Egypt, South America, and Taiwan vary somewhat on which patients are considered older and the applicable treatment target for the population.[24] The older population is considered to be anywhere from 60 years to 80 years and older. Target blood pressure ranges from greater than 140/90, generally for patients ≥65 years, to less than 150/90 for those ≥80 years.[24] The European Society of Hypertension/European Society of Cardiology Guidelines specifically highlighted that whether older patients with blood pressure between 140 and 160 mm Hg should be treated is still a significant gap in the literature.[19] As mentioned, other reviews and consensus panels have also specifically stated that the management of HTN in people 80 and older is still uncertain.

One challenge is the existing guidelines do not suggest the minimal level above which a blood pressure should be controlled, whether for systolic or diastolic pressure.[25] Studies suggest a J-shaped or U-shaped curve in the associations between blood pressure and cardiovascular outcomes, with a nadir for risk at 135/75 mm Hg in people 70 to 79 and 140/70 for people ≥80 years.[6] However, concerns regarding this association between BP and risk include the methodologic quality of studies showing the association and the lack of consideration of confounders like heart failure, age, and comorbidity. One suggestion is that wide pulse pressure and low DBP are more important risk predictors that may be related to the J-curve association.[26] Although some recommendations are to increase the goal SBP to less than 150 mm Hg for the older population to avoid harms, there is still a lack of definitive evidence and a lack of agreement among experts.[25] The evidence is particularly uncertain for higher risk groups, particularly with cardiovascular disease, multiple risk factors, and African Americans who may have a higher risk of morbidity and mortality using higher SBP targets and who may benefit from more aggressive treatment goals.[7]

UNIQUE ISSUES IN THE ELDERLY POPULATION
Frailty

Little is known about the treatment of hypertension in frail older persons. Other than studies in long-term care settings, studies of antihypertensive treatment have not specifically focused on frail individuals to test hypotheses about benefits and harms of overtreatment or undertreatment in the context of frailty.[27] The HYVET trial did include a 25-item frailty index, and a secondary study of participants for whom there was frailty data found no interaction between frailty and benefits or harms in the study.[28] Frail and fit participants both seemed to benefit from blood pressure reduction. In the SPRINT trial, frailty was characterized using a 36-item Frailty Index. For every 1% increase in the Frailty Index, there was a higher risk of injurious falls with a hazard ratio of 1.035, and increased risk of all-cause hospitalizations with a hazard ratio of 1.038.[29]

However, findings regarding the harms of antihypertensive therapy in nursing home settings do raise concern for the potential for overtreatment in frail older persons. In the Predictive Values of Blood Pressure and Arterial Stiffness in Institutionalized Very Aged Population (PARTAGE) study, there was a higher risk of all-cause mortality in patients with SBP less than 130 mm Hg taking 2 or more antihypertensive medications. The authors recommended that people 80 and older who are considered robust by a rapid frailty assessment could be treated with a similar approach to patients aged 65 to 75 years, with a target SBP 130 to 150 mm Hg. For frail individuals, target SBP should be 150 mm Hg, and HTN should be treated with monotherapy at low dose, with slow dosage increases, and with a reduction in therapy if patients have SBP less than 130 mm Hg or orthostatic hypotension.[30]

Cognition

The American Heart Association released a consensus statement in October 2016 that although there is a clear adverse effect of midlife hypertension on late-life cognitive function, there is not enough evidence to make recommendations about late-life hypertension and late-life cognitive impairment. Furthermore, in the oldest patients ($\geq$85 years) there is even less evidence, with a suggestion that higher SBP was associated with better cognitive function and other data suggesting that hypertension might be associated with other cognitive dysfunction but not with short-term memory loss.[31] A cohort study of patients 75 and older showed that higher SBP was associated with lower mortality in patients with cognitive and functional impairment.[32] However, discontinuing antihypertensive medications in patients 75 and older with mild cognitive impairment did not result in any improvements in cognitive, psychological, or functional ability.[33]

Stroke

HTN is the most important modifiable risk factor for both hemorrhagic and ischemic stroke in adults. Isolated systolic HTN and elevated pulse pressures are significantly more important estimations of elevated stroke risk compared with diastolic pressures.[34]

Diastolic pressures pushed low by attempts to treat isolated systolic HTN were once thought to result in hypoperfusion to the brain and increased stroke risk in older adults. Although diastolic pressures $\leq$60 mm Hg can result in other cardiovascular events, this finding does not correlate to increased incidence of stroke.[35,36] This creates a therapeutic range in which to keep pressures neither too high nor too low to maximize outcomes including stroke.

SUMMARY

Hypertension remains a common problem among elderly patients. Although much data has been accumulated in the last several years about both the measurement and treatment of HTN including elderly patients, confusion about whom to treat and how low to drive pressures has continued to be a difficulty for providers. The basic principles, however, remain the same for elderly patients. For older community-living younger elders (<80 years of age), treatment should follow that of other adults. These younger, more functional geriatric patients can often be driven to goal blood pressure reductions to maximize their outcomes. As physiologic reserve declines and patients become frail, these patients are not able to compensate for lower reductions in blood pressures. This inability to compensate can result in hypoperfusion of the heart and brain and subsequent increased incidence of heart attack and stroke. Additionally, medications used to lower blood pressures as well as the low pressures themselves have a significant effect on patient's quality of life, causing dizziness, falls, and fatigue.

Focusing on individual patient goals and tolerability is important in the treatment of all patients but is crucial to the treatment of older or frail patients. Providers should focus on goals of care discussions and quality of life before starting medications or other aggressive interventions in frail and elderly patients. When medications are initiated, patients should be started on low doses, taking care to choose medications less likely to cause excessive lowering of blood pressure or orthostatic hypotension. Patients should be advised of possible side effects and should follow up with practitioners routinely.

REFERENCES

1. Egan BM, Zhao Y, Axon RN. US trends in prevalence, awareness, treatment, and control of hypertension, 1988-2008. JAMA 2010;303(20):2043–50.
2. Wright JD, Hughes JP, Ostchega Y, et al. Mean systolic and diastolic blood pressure in adults aged 18 and over in the United States, 2001-2008. Natl Health Stat Report 2011;(35):1–22, 24.
3. Dai X, Hummel SL, Salazar JB, et al. Cardiovascular physiology in the older adults. J Geriatr Cardiol 2015;12(3):196–201.
4. Franklin SS, Larson MG, Khan SA, et al. Does the relation of blood pressure to coronary heart disease risk change with aging? The Framingham Heart Study. Circulation 2001;103(9):1245–9.
5. Kaplan NM, Victor RG. Hypertension in the Population at Large. In: Kaplan NM, Victor RG, editors. Kaplan's clinical hypertension. 11th edition. Philadelphia: Wolters Kluwer; 2014. p. 1–17.
6. Aronow WS, Fleg JL, Pepine CJ, et al. ACCF/AHA 2011 expert consensus document on hypertension in the elderly: a report of the American College of Cardiology Foundation Task Force on clinical expert consensus documents developed in collaboration with the American Academy of Neurology, American Geriatrics Society, American Society for Preventive Cardiology, American Society of Hypertension, American Society of Nephrology, Association of Black Cardiologists, and European Society of Hypertension. J Am Soc Hypertens 2011;5(4):259–352.
7. Siu AL. Screening for high blood pressure in adults: U.S. Preventive Services Task Force recommendation statement. Ann Intern Med 2015;163(10):778–86.
8. James PA, Oparil S, Carter BL, et al. 2014 evidence-based guideline for the management of high blood pressure in adults: report from the panel members appointed to the Eighth Joint National Committee (JNC 8). JAMA 2014;311(5):507–20.
9. Petersen ME, Williams TR, Gordon C, et al. The normal response to prolonged passive head up tilt testing. Heart 2000;84:509–14.
10. Consensus statement on the definition of orthostatic hypotension, pure autonomic failure, and multiple system atrophy. The Consensus Committee of the American Autonomic Society and the American Academy of Neurology. Neurology 1996;46:1470.
11. Ooi WL, Barrett S, Hossain M, et al. Patterns of orthostatic blood pressure change and their clinical correlates in a frail, elderly population. JAMA 1997;277:1299–304.
12. Lipsitz LA. Orthostatic hypotension in the elderly. N Engl J Med 1989;321:952–7.
13. Wolters FJ, Mattace-Raso FU, Koudstaal PJ, et al. Orthostatic hypotension and the long-term risk of dementia: a population-based study. PLoS Med 2016;13(10):e1002143.
14. Kohler S, Baars MA, Spauwen P, et al. Temporal evolution of cognitive changes in incident hypertension: prospective cohort study across the adult age span. Hypertension 2014;63:245–51.

15. Gottesman RF, Schneider AL, Albert M, et al. Midlife hypertension and 20-year cognitive change: the atherosclerosis risk in communities neurocognitive study. JAMA Neurol 2014;71(10):1218–27.
16. Musini VM, Tejani AM, Bassett K, et al. Pharmacotherapy for hypertension in the elderly. Cochrane Database Syst Rev 2009;(4):CD000028.
17. Aronow WS. Treating hypertension and prehypertension in older people: when, whom and how. Maturitas 2015;80(1):31–6.
18. National Institute for Health and Care Excellence Hypertension Pathway. Available at: https://pathways.nice.org.uk/pathways/hypertension. Accessed October 27, 2016.
19. Mancia G, Fagard R, Narkiewicz K, et al. 2013 ESH/ESC guidelines for the management of arterial hypertension: the Task Force for the Management of Arterial Hypertension of the European Society of Hypertension (ESH) and of the European Society of Cardiology (ESC). Eur Heart J 2013;34(28):2159–219.
20. Buford TW. Hypertension and aging. Ageing Res Rev 2016;26:96–111.
21. Wright JT Jr, Williamson JD, Whelton PK, et al. A randomized trial of intensive versus standard blood-pressure control. N Engl J Med 2015;373(22):2103–16.
22. Williamson JD, Supiano MA, Applegate WB, et al. Intensive vs standard blood pressure control and cardiovascular disease outcomes in adults aged >/=75 years: a randomized clinical trial. JAMA 2016;315(24):2673–82.
23. Bress AP, Tanner RM, Hess R, et al. Generalizability of SPRINT results to the U.S. adult population. J Am Coll Cardiol 2016;67(5):463–72.
24. Alhawassi TM, Krass I, Pont LG. Hypertension in older persons: a systematic review of national and international treatment guidelines. J Clin Hypertens (Greenwich) 2015;17(6):486–92.
25. Jansen J, McKinn S, Bonner C, et al. Systematic review of clinical practice guidelines recommendations about primary cardiovascular disease prevention for older adults. BMC Fam Pract 2015;16:104.
26. Rosendorff C, Lackland DT, Allison M, et al. Treatment of hypertension in patients with coronary artery disease: a scientific statement from the American Heart Association, American College of Cardiology, and American Society of Hypertension. Circulation 2015;131(19):e435–470.
27. Materson BJ, Garcia-Estrada M, Preston RA. Hypertension in the frail elderly. J Am Soc Hypertens 2016;10(6):536–41.
28. Warwick J, Falaschetti E, Rockwood K, et al. No evidence that frailty modifies the positive impact of antihypertensive treatment in very elderly people: an investigation of the impact of frailty upon treatment effect in the HYpertension in the Very Elderly Trial (HYVET) study, a double-blind, placebo-controlled study of antihypertensives in people with hypertension aged 80 and over. BMC Med 2015; 13:78.
29. Pajewski NM, Williamson JD, Applegate WB, et al. Characterizing frailty status in the systolic blood pressure intervention trial. J Gerontol A Biol Sci Med Sci 2016; 71(5):649–55.
30. Benetos A, Rossignol P, Cherubini A, et al. Polypharmacy in the aging patient: management of hypertension in octogenarians. JAMA 2015;314(2):170–80.
31. Iadecola C, Yaffe K, Biller J, et al. Impact of hypertension on cognitive function: a scientific statement from the American Heart Association. Hypertension 2016; 68(6):e67–94.
32. Oliva RV, Bakris GL. Management of hypertension in the elderly population. J Gerontol A Biol Sci Med Sci 2012;67(12):1343–51.

33. Moonen JEF, Foster-Dingley JC, de Ruijter W, et al. Effect of discontinuation of antihypertensive treatment in elderly people on cognitive functioning—the DANTE study leiden: a randomized clinical trial. JAMA Intern Med 2015; 175(10):1622.
34. Mozaffarian D, Benjamin EJ, Go AS, et al. Heart disease and stroke statistics-2016 update: a report from the American Heart Association. Circulation 2016; 133(4):e38–360.
35. Protogerou AD, Safar ME, Iaria P, et al. Diastolic blood pressure and mortality in the elderly with cardiovascular disease. Hypertension 2007;50(1):172–80.
36. Bangalore S, Messerli FH, Wun CC, et al. J-curve revisited: an analysis of blood pressure and cardiovascular events in the treating to new targets (TNT) trial. Eur Heart J 2010;31(23):2897–908.

Delirium

Belinda Setters, MD, MS[a,b,*], Laurence M. Solberg, MD[c]

KEYWORDS

- Delirium • Encephalopathy • Acute mental status change • Confusion • Elderly

KEY POINTS

- Delirium is a geriatric syndrome characterized by acute confusion and inattention that may persist in a subacute form lasting for weeks or even months.
- Delirium is a manifestation of an underlying condition and is often considered multifactorial. Common causes in elderly patients include infections, urinary retention, pain, and medication side effects. Finding and treating the underlying causes are key to resolving delirium.
- Delirium has significant morbidity and mortality. It not only increases risk of falls and prolonged hospitalization, it may result in irreversible cognitive decline and even death.
- Because of its association with dementia and poor outcomes, delirium is an important geriatric syndrome for primary care providers to know as they care for an increasing geriatric population.

INTRODUCTION

Delirium is a common neurocognitive disorder characterized by an acute change in cognition, attention, and consciousness that results in what experts describe as brain failure. Delirium has traditionally been discussed in the acute-care setting, where it occurs in up to 80% of patients.[1] Despite much lower incidence of delirium in outpatient care areas, population aging makes it more likely that primary care providers will encounter patients with delirium. These trends, combined with delirium's high morbidity and mortality, make delirium an important topic that primary providers should not ignore.

Delirium is known by a variety of different terms, including altered mental status, acute mental status change, encephalopathy, agitation, altered level of consciousness,

No Disclosures.
[a] Department of Internal Medicine, Robley Rex VAMC, University of Louisville, 800 Zorn Avenue, 6 West – GEC #627, Louisville, KY 40206, USA; [b] Inpatient Geriatrics, Department of Family & Geriatric Medicine, Robley Rex VAMC, University of Louisville, 800 Zorn Avenue, 6 West – GEC #627, Louisville, KY 40206, USA; [c] GRECC, Division of Geriatric Medicine, Department of Aging and Geriatric Research, Malcom Randall VAMC, University of Florida College of Medicine, 2004 Mowry Road, Gainesville, FL 32610, USA
* Corresponding author. Department of Internal Medicine, Robley Rex VAMC, University of Louisville, 800 Zorn Avenue, 6 West – GEC #627, Louisville, KY 40206.
E-mail address: belinda.setters@va.gov

Prim Care Clin Office Pract 44 (2017) 541–559
http://dx.doi.org/10.1016/j.pop.2017.04.010
0095-4543/17/© 2017 Elsevier Inc. All rights reserved.
primarycare.theclinics.com

brain failure, and even psychosis. Although these terms are descriptive of symptoms, the ongoing use of so many different terms can be confusing to trainees, providers, and families. In addition, the lack of a clear pathologic process and the slowness of many practitioners to adopt validated diagnostic methods has resulted in continued underdiagnosis.[2]

Delirium has been vaguely described for more than 2 centuries, but it has only been formally defined since the mid-1990s by the American Psychiatric Association's Diagnostic and Statistical Manual of Mental Disorders, Fourth Edition (DMS-IV). Earlier editions described organic psychosis symptoms, whereas later editions (DSM-IV and DSM-V) describe it more specifically as an acute change in mental status with a fluctuating course, inattention, disturbance of consciousness, and disorganized thinking.[3] The DSM has become the gold standard from which various screens and assessment criteria have been formulated in an effort to make bedside diagnosis easier and more efficient.

Delirium is not only common but also has a significant health care burden. Although 30% to 40% is preventable,[4–6] once it occurs, delirium results in increased debility and loss of function as well as increased morbidity and mortality and health care costs,[7–12] making it a significant public health burden costing more than $164 billion annually in the United States alone.[12]

EPIDEMIOLOGY

The overall prevalence of delirium varies widely, between 9% and 80% by setting, with lower levels among outpatient and residential care homes.[1,10–13] The lowest incidence occurs in the outpatient office setting, at only 2%,[10,13] but this is expected to increase with population aging and age-associated increases in multimorbidity and dementia.[14,15] In addition, patients presenting with delirium almost always require emergency medical care or hospital admission. Among elderly patients presenting to emergency departments (EDs), up to 17% of all community-dwelling seniors and 40% of nursing home residents present with this diagnosis.[16]

Patients requiring hospital admission, between 18% and 35% of patients had a diagnosis of delirium on admission.[1,16] Once hospitalized, elderly patients have a high risk of developing delirium, especially if they have an underlying dementia disorder. Those in postoperative wards, intensive care units (ICUs), geriatric wards, and hospice wards had the highest prevalence of delirium 50% to 80%.[10,11,13,16,17] Delirium is also prevalent in the skilled nursing facilities and postacute care (PAC) settings after discharge from acute hospitalization, with more than 9% of patients having documented evidence of delirium on admission to PAC facilities.[18] This situation leads to an overall delirium rate of 29% to 64% for older adult patients.[1]

Patients who develop delirium are at increased risk for a variety of poor outcomes, including falls, catheter-associated infections, and debility, as well as prolonged hospital stay, and increased likelihood of physical restraints and antipsychotic medication administration. Patients who develop delirium in the ICU are at 2 to 4 times increased risk for death both during and after hospitalization[13,19,20]; those on general medicine or surgical wards have a 1.5-fold increased risk of death in the year after hospitalization.[21–23] Patients visiting the ED who are diagnosed with delirium have up to 70% increased risk of death in the first 6 months after their visit.[24]

Aging

Although cognitive loss is not a normal aging phenomenon, the development of cognitive loss such as dementia occurs more commonly with aging. Autopsy studies indicate that as many as half of all older adults (>80 years old) have changes consistent with Alzheimer disease at death.[25,26] As previously mentioned, with the aging population and increasing rates of multimorbidity, more patients will be living longer with precursor risks for dementia and therefore delirium.[14,15] Primary care providers will be expected to care for more older patients with dementia and therefore delirium.

It is common for patients with undiagnosed dementia to be diagnosed with delirium while hospitalized or acutely ill. Delirium in patients without a previous diagnosis of dementia may be a red flag to suggest underlying cognitive loss.[27,28] In addition, patients with dementia have more significant decline when they develop delirium compared with patients with no underlying cognitive deficits.[29–32] Preexisting cognitive disorders lower the threshold for delirium. This is why patients with dementia are more prone to develop delirium from what would otherwise be an uncomplicated urinary tract infection. Unfortunately, delirium can result in cognitive impairment like dementia in patients without prior cognitive deficits.[33]

ASSESSMENT

Delirium is diagnosed clinically as there are currently no laboratory or radiological studies available to confirm its presence. Most physicians find the DSM cumbersome and time consuming as they are not trained in its use and have increasingly limited time with patients. To combat this problem, several diagnostic tools have been developed to allow clinicians to diagnose delirium more efficiently and effectively.[34]

Similarly educating nurses to identify delirium has been shown to be effective as nurses in acute and post-acute care settings have more contact with the patients on a daily basis than physicians.[35] Screening tests such as the Nursing Delirium Screening scale (Nu-DESC), Delirium Observational Screening scale (DOS), and NEECHAM have been used to evaluate delirium risk, but are not diagnostic.[36–38] They are mostly used by nursing staff to predict individual patients' risks for developing delirium in the acute-care setting. However, tools such as the confusion assessment method (CAM)[39] and the 4-AT[40] useful in diagnosing delirium. The CAM is the most commonly used tool, especially in its short form, which simplifies its use at the bedside.[41] The 4-AT in the U.S., a newer tool, is also gaining acceptance especially in the U.K. where it was developed. **Fig. 1** shows the flow used

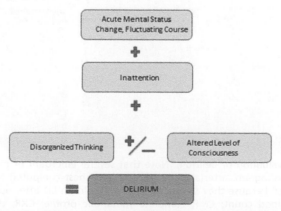

Fig. 1. CAM criteria for delirium diagnosis. (*Data from* Inouye SK. Short CAM: Training manual and Coding Guide. 2014; Boston: Hospital Elder Life Program.)

by the CAM short form. The CAM can be accessed at www.hospitalelderlifeprogram. org and the 4-AT at www.scottishdeliriumassociation.com. The 4-AT can also be viewed in Appendix 1.

In addition to the original and short versions of the CAM, an ICU version[42,43] has been validated specifically for use in critical care wards and EDs. The use of a tool is very important in diagnosing delirium regardless of which one is used. Research has shown that providers lack knowledge of delirium and underdiagnose when tools are not used.[44–46]

Identification of an organic underlying cause is also important in diagnosing and treating delirium.[47] Identifying an underlying organic cause helps differentiate delirium from psychosis, a non-organic, psychiatric disorder. This distinction also helps distinguish the behavioral disturbances often associated with dementia from delirium. Pearls for evaluation are listed in **Fig. 2**.

Careful review of the diagnostic criteria of delirium aids in making this distinction. Although patients with dementia may be confused, their confusion should not occur

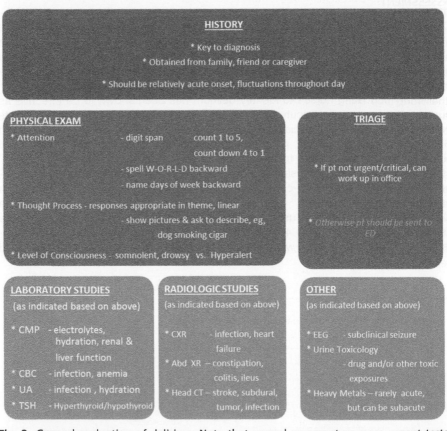

Fig. 2. General evaluation of delirium. Note that several emergent or more urgent tests, such as electrocardiogram, arterial blood draws, and chest computed tomography (CT), have been omitted because they should be performed in an ED after appropriate triage. CBC, complete blood count; CMP, complete metabolic profile; CXR, chest radiograph; EEG, electroencephalogram; pt, patient; TSH, thyroid-stimulating hormone; UA, urinalysis; XR, radiograph.

acutely nor should it have a fluctuating course. The exception to this is Lewy body dementia, which can have fluctuations in course as well as inattention.[48] However, patients with dementia can hold attention and organize their thoughts, compared with delirious patients who cannot. Care should be taken in making this distinction in the outpatient office. Delirium should be considered an urgent, if not emergent, situation requiring appropriate triage and referral.

PATHOPHYSIOLOGY

The pathophysiology of delirium is extremely complex and still not well understood. Each individual patient with delirium has a unique set of underlying causes contributing to their symptoms.[49–51] The interplay between a patient's existing pathophysiology and the changes occurring with an acute illness result in an imbalance of brain chemistry. Although the individual predisposing factors, acute illness, pathways, and chemicals involved may vary, the result is the same, acute brain failure. Factors involved in delirium pathophysiology can be separated into preexisting risk factors and predisposing actors which are listed in **Table 1**.

Older patients, especially those over 80 years old, are at increased risk, as are patients with genetic predispositions. Although the genetic predispositions are not well known, age seems to predispose to delirium development in its association with an increased incidence of dementia.[32,33] As a cohort, older patients also have more comorbidities as a cohort compared with younger patients and therefore take more medications. The increased burden of adverse side effects and the number of medications taken has also been shown to contribute to delirium occurrence.[51–55]

Metabolic derangements are common causes of delirium.[49,56] Alterations in electrolytes such as sodium and potassium, as well as glucose imbalances, are commonly seen in this role. Dehydration, uremia, and hepatic dysfunction also contribute to delirium, as does hypoxia and hypercapnia.[49,56,57] Some of these factors, like glucose, directly affect the brain's ability to function, whereas others, like dehydration and inflammatory cascades, work more indirectly.[58–60] Inflammation works this way by causing cytokine activation, which in turn leads to impaired blood flow and neuronal death.[61,62] Likewise, infection causing inflammatory cascades and impaired flow leads to delirium.[63,64]

Table 1
Common factors in the development of delirium

Risk Factors	Precipitating Factors
Advanced age	Polypharmacy (≥5 medications)
Cognitive impairment, dementia	Psychoactive or sedative medications
Functional impairment, debility	Infection
Sensory impairment, hearing and visual loss	Surgery or trauma
Transient ischemic attack, stroke	Indwelling urinary catheter
Alcohol dependence, abuse	Physical restraints
Major depression	Coma
Comorbidity level, complex multimorbidity	Physiologic/metabolic derangements (abnormal blood urea nitrogen/creatinine, urea, pH, sodium, glucose)

Neurotransmitters such as acetylcholine, serotonin, gamma-aminobutyric acid, and dopamine become imbalanced in delirium, which results in the inability of delirious patients to process information and respond appropriately, as shown in **Fig. 3**.[65,66] The result is the clinical manifestation of delirium, an acute confusional state with the inability to hold attention. Thought processes are typically disorganized and the level of consciousness is often affected. As a result, patients are typically either hypervigilant or somnolent, at times appearing almost comatose. Delirium can occur in a mixed state as well, alternating between an agitated, hypervigilant state and a somnolent, hypoalert one. These fluctuations form the types of delirium: hyperactive, hypoactive and mixed.[67]

Older patients accumulate neuronal, dendritic, and microglial damage or even death over time.[65] They are also more likely to have cerebrovascular disease and a history of head trauma. As a result, older brains seem to be less able to deal with stressors and more likely to develop and have difficulty clearing delirium.

Causes

As mentioned earlier, most cases of delirium result from a complex multifactorial process[49,65] (**Fig. 4**). It is important to determine underlying causes contributing to this syndrome since treating these issues is the best way to clear delirium.

Neurologic conditions such as stroke, encephalitis or meningitis, and ischemic or traumatic brain injury are obvious potential causes of delirium. Cardiovascular disorders that impair blood flow and oxygenation are also important causes, including myocardial infarction, heart failure, pulmonary embolism, and shock. Infections can cause delirium with urinary tract infections and pneumonia being the most common among older patients.

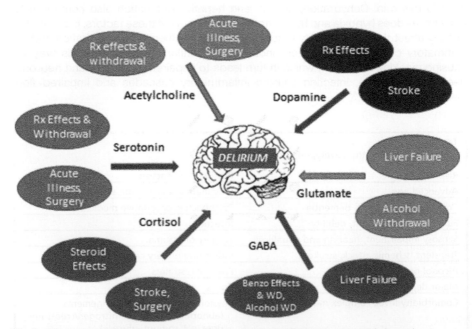

Fig. 3. Neurotransmitter imbalance in delirium. Rx, medication; WD, withdrawal.

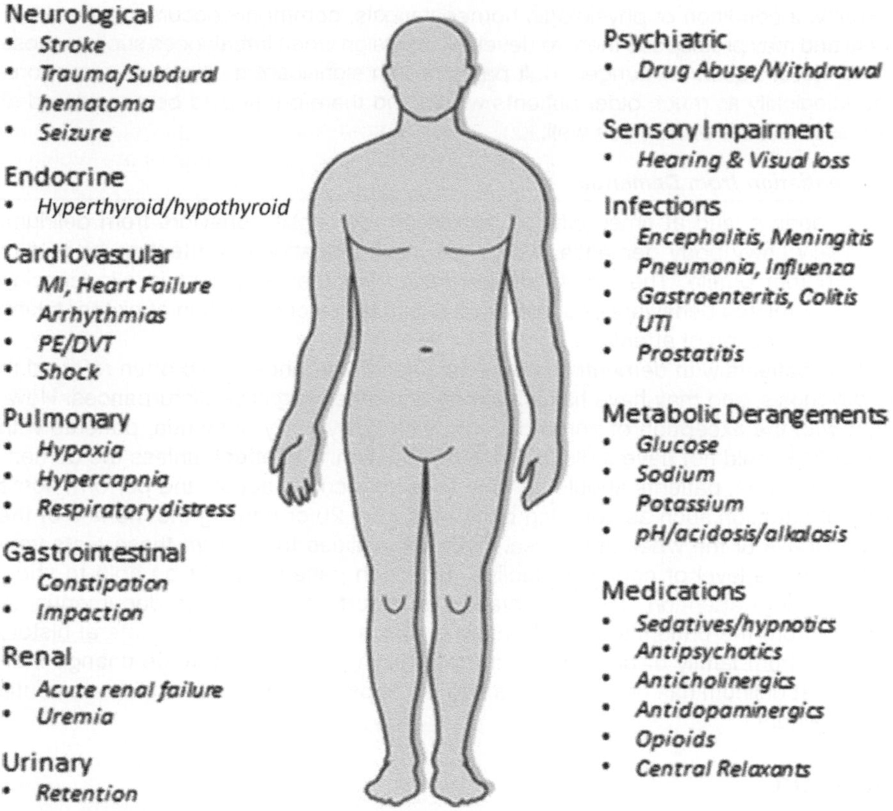

Neurological
* Stroke
* Trauma/Subdural hematoma
* Seizure

Endocrine
* Hyperthyroid/hypothyroid

Cardiovascular
* MI, Heart Failure
* Arrhythmias
* PE/DVT
* Shock

Pulmonary
* Hypoxia
* Hypercapnia
* Respiratory distress

Gastrointestinal
* Constipation
* Impaction

Renal
* Acute renal failure
* Uremia

Urinary
* Retention

Psychiatric
* Drug Abuse/Withdrawal

Sensory Impairment
* Hearing & Visual loss

Infections
* Encephalitis, Meningitis
* Pneumonia, Influenza
* Gastroenteritis, Colitis
* UTI
* Prostatitis

Metabolic Derangements
* Glucose
* Sodium
* Potassium
* pH/acidosis/alkalosis

Medications
* Sedatives/hypnotics
* Antipsychotics
* Anticholinergics
* Antidopaminergics
* Opioids
* Central Relaxants

Fig. 4. Common causes of delirium by system. MI, myocardial infarction; PE/DVT, pulmonary embolism/deep vein thrombosis; UTI, urinary tract infection.

Age related changes predispose older adults to have difficulty emptying the bladder and rectum. Sarcopenia, the systemic loss of skeletal and smooth muscle that occurs with more advanced aging, contributes to these disorders, making urinary retention and constipation/impaction common causes of delirium in this population.

Pain is another cause of delirium that practitioners do not want to miss. Uncontrolled pain causes significant distress and, if untreated, can result in delirium. Detecting pain among elderly patients can be more difficult because of sensory loss, communication difficulties, stoicism and dementia. Cognitively impaired patients must be especially watched for nonverbal signs of pain because they cannot reliably report their pain symptoms.

Medication side effects and toxins, including heavy metals, can also cause delirium.[51,55] Although almost any medication or herbal remedy can cause delirium, some drug classes have been clearly shown to be more likely to do so. These drugs include anticholinergic medications, antidopaminergics, antipsychotics, hypnotics, and sedatives, as well as other centrally acting drugs.[52–55] Medications have been assessed through a variety of ways to assist clinicians in gauging which medications are less likely to cause confusion in elderly or at-risk patients, such as the Beers criteria[68] and the Anticholinergic Burden Score.[69,70] Some common medications known to cause delirium are listed in **Table 2**. Note that herbals and over-the-counter medications.

Frailty, a condition of physiologic homeostenosis, commonly occurs in elderly patients and may predispose them to develop confusion when imbalances such as those noted earlier occur.[71] Younger adult patients with significant multimorbidity respond physiologically as much older patients would and therefore should be considered at increased risk for delirium as well.

Differentiation from Dementia

It is important, and at times difficult, to discern dementia behaviors from delirium, especially Lewy body dementia, which can have alterations in attention as part of its symptom profile. The key to differentiating whether a patient is experiencing dementia-related behaviors or acute brain failure is in a combination of history taking and determination of attention.

Many patients with dementia have behavioral disturbances, also often referred to as psychosis, and may have hallucinations and other cognitive disturbances. However, with the exception of some patients with Lewy body dementia, patients with dementia should not have a disturbance of attention.[48] In effect, unless the dementia is end stage, patients should be able to have a conversation and perform some tests of attention such as counting backward from 20 or naming the months of the year or days of the week in reverse. Patients' abilities to perform these tests vary based on the level of cognitive decline, but each patient should be able to show some level of attention. This observation is important, along with documenting a change from the patient's normal baseline status (obtained from collateral history obtained from family or caregivers), in determining whether an acute change indicates that delirium has occurred. This finding helps clinicians differentiate dementia from delirium.

TREATMENT

Delirium treatment should focus on addressing the underlying cause (**Fig. 5**). Treating the cause for brain failure is the only way to achieve clearing of delirium. Many studies have attempted to address prevention as well as treatment of behavioral disturbances, including agitation, that can be associated with delirium.

Identification of at-risk populations of patients should be part of hospital admissions as well as provider assessments in all care areas. The following precipitating factors

Table 2
Common medications that cause delirium

Drug Class	Example Medications
Anticholinergics	Diphenhydramine, promethazine, oxybutynin
Antidopaminergics	Metocloperamide, chlorpromazine, bupropion
Sedative/hypnotics	Benzodiazepines: diazepam, clonazepam Barbiturates: secobarbital, phenobarbital Hypnotics: zolpidem, zaleplon, ramelteon
Antipsychotics	Haloperidol, quetiapine, olanzapine, ziprasidone
Opioids	Hydrocodone, oxycodone, morphine
Other centrally acting agents	Relaxants: tizanidine, cyclobenzaprine, baclofen Dopaminergic: carbidopa/levodopa, selegiline Stimulants: amphetamine, methylphenidate

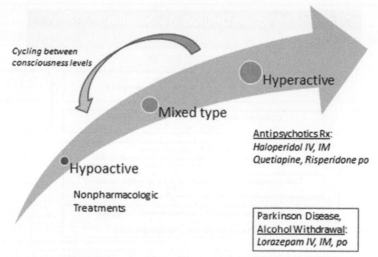

Fig. 5. Delirium treatment by type. IM, intramuscular; IV, intravenous; po, by mouth.

should be considered when assessing for delirium risk: cognitive impairment and disorientation, dehydration, hypoxia, immobility, infection, polypharmacy, pain, malnutrition, sensory impairment, and sleep disturbance.[72] Education of health care providers on the recognition of risks and symptoms of delirium has been shown to reduce the prevalence.[73–78]

Treatment guidelines for both hyperactive and hypoactive delirium recommend avoidance of medications, including sedatives and antipsychotics, in favor of nonpharmacologic interventions because there is no clear evidence for the use of these medications in delirium.[47,79,80] Supportive care by family members and nursing should focus on close, continuing observation.[81,82] Reassuring patients that they are safe, and reorientating them to place, people, and plans are also helpful.[47] Pharmacologic interventions should be reserved for the management of persistent behavioral symptoms that do not respond to nonpharmacologic treatments and place the patient at risk for harming themselves or others.[81,83–86]

Many practitioners still use antipsychotic medications for both hyperactive and hypoactive delirium despite the lack of clear evidence to support their use.[85] Haloperidol has long been considered the gold standard medication for the treatment of persistent agitated behaviors not responsive to nonpharmacologic interventions. It remains the most commonly used medication despite waning evidence for its efficacy in either prevention or treatment of delirium.[84,85]

More recently, newer second-generation antipsychotics such as quetiapine, risperidone, and olanzapine have been used for short-term treatment in patients who are able and/or agreeable to take oral medications. However, olanzapine is the only one to be included in prior recommendations.[83] When these medications are used, practitioners should be cautioned to ensure that corrected QT (QTc) (per 12-lead electrocardiogram) is not prolonged because antipsychotic medications are known to cause prolongation. In addition, a thorough medication review should be done to ensure there are no potential drug interactions or other medications that might contribute to prolongation of the QTc.[83,87]

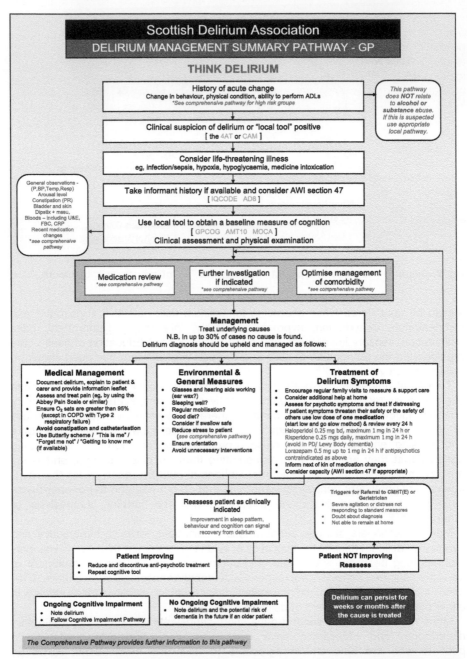

Fig. 6. Scottish Delirium Association delirium management summary pathway. ADLs, activities of daily living; BP, blood pressure; COPD, chronic obstructive pulmonary disease; CRP, C-reactive protein; GP, general practitioner; P, pulse; Resp, respiration; Temp, temperature. (*From* Scottish Delirium Association. Available at: http://www.scottishdeliriumassociation. com/. Accessed February 10, 2017; with permission.)

In general, benzodiazepine medication should be avoided for most patients because these medications can worsen delirium.[88] For some patients who have persistent, resistant symptoms, or specialized groups such as patients experiencing alcohol or benzodiazepine withdrawal or patients with Parkinson disease, these medications may be used at the discretion of the practitioner and assuming that the risks are outweighed by potential benefits of the medication. As with all medication dosing in the elderly, benzodiazepine and antipsychotic doses should be low and initiated cautiously.

Guideline flow charts such as those published by the Scottish Delirium Society (scottishdelirium.com) help simplify the complexity of addressing delirium assessment and treatment. The chart for general practitioners is shown in **Fig. 6**. Additional guidelines for nursing homes and a more comprehensive guideline can be found in Appendices 2 and 3.

SUMMARY

Although delirium remains primarily an acute-care issue, its importance cannot be overestimated for primary care, outpatient specialty, postacute care, and long-term care providers. With the continued aging of the world population, dementia, and with it delirium, will continue to be common health problems. Prompt identification of delirium and its differentiation from dementia will be important to quickly discern necessary treatment in the outpatient setting. This distinction includes knowing when to refer patients for emergency or inpatient care. Likewise, learning to identify prolonged or subacute delirium in patients recently hospitalized will be important for outpatient providers. As research continues in delirium, providers will be able to better avoid precipitating factors such as offending medications while providing more specific treatments to clear this important geriatric syndrome.

REFERENCES

1. Inouye SK, Westendorp RG, Saczynski JS. Delirium in elderly people. Lancet 2014;383:911–22.
2. Inouye SK. Delirium in older persons. N Engl J Med 2006;354:1157–65.
3. American Psychiatric Association. Diagnostic and statistical manual of mental disorders. 5th edition. Washington (DC): American Psychiatric Association; 2013.
4. Inouye SK, Bogardus ST Jr, Charpentier PA, et al. A multicomponent intervention to prevent delirium in hospitalized older patients. N Engl J Med 1999;340:669–76.
5. Marcantonio ER, Flacker JM, Wright RJ, et al. Reducing delirium after hip fracture: a randomized trial. J Am Geriatr Soc 2001;49:516–22.
6. O'Mahony R, Murthy L, Akunne A, et al. Synopsis of the National Institute for Health and Clinical Excellence guideline for prevention of delirium. Ann Intern Med 2011;154:746–51.
7. Inouye SK, Rushing JT, Foreman MD, et al. Does delirium contribute to poor hospital outcomes? a three-site epidemiologic study. J Gen Intern Med 1998;13: 234–42.
8. Murray AM, Levkoff SE, Wetle TT, et al. Acute delirium and functional decline in the hospitalized elderly patient. J Gerontol 1993;48:M181–6.
9. Pompei P, Foreman M, Rudberg MA, et al. Delirium in hospitalized older persons: outcome and predictors. J Am Geriatr Soc 1994;42:809–15.

10. Siddiqui N, House AO, Holmes JD. Occurrence and outcome of delirium in medical in-patients: a systemic literature review. Age Ageing 2006;35: 350–64.
11. Brummel NE, Jackson JCP, Pandharipande PP, et al. Delirium in the ICU and subsequent long-term disability among survivors of mechanical ventilation. Crit Care Med 2014;42(2):369–77.
12. Leslie DL, Marcantionio ER, Zhang Y, et al. One-year health care costs associated with delirium in the elderly population. Arch Intern Med 2008;168(1): 27–32.
13. Van den Boogaard M, Schoonhoven L, van der Hoeven LG, et al. Incidence and short-term consequences of delirium in critically ill patients: a prospective observational cohort study. Int J Nurs Stud 2012;49:775–83.
14. Hebert LE, Weuve J, Scherr PA, et al. Alzheimer's disease in the United States (2010-2050) estimated using the 2010 census. Neurology 2013;80: 1778–83.
15. Jacqmin-Gadda H, Alperovitch A, Monlahuc D, et al. 20-year prevalence projections for dementia and impact of preventive policy about risk factors. Eur J Epidemiol 2013;28:493–502.
16. Qian X, Russell LB, Valiyeva E, et al. "Quicker and sicker" under Medicare's prospective payment system for hospitals: new evidence on an old issue from a national longitudinal survey. Bull Econ Res 2011;63(1):1–27.
17. Hill TE, Osterweil D, Bakerjian D, et al. "Post-acute care 2.0" regarding, Burke RE, Whitfield EA, Hittle D, et al. Hospital readmission from post-acute care facilities: risk factors, timing, and outcomes. J Am Med Dir Assoc 2016;17(4): 368–9.
18. Morandi A, Solberg LM, Habermann R, et al. Documentation and management of words associated with delirium among elderly patients in postacute care: a pilot investigation. J Am Med Dir Assoc 2009;10(5):330–4.
19. Jones RN, Kiely DK, Marcantonio ER. Prevalence of delirium on admission to post-acute care is associated with higher number of nursing home deficiencies. J Am Med Dir Assoc 2010;11(4):253–6.
20. Francis J. Delirium in older patients. J Am Geriatr Soc 1992;40(8):829–38.
21. Hosie A, Davidson PM, Agar M, et al. Delirium prevalence, incidence, and implications for screening in specialist palliative care inpatient settings: a systematic review. Palliat Med 2013;27:486–98.
22. Ely EW, Shintani A, Truman B, et al. Delirium as a predictor of mortality in mechanically ventilated patients in the intensive care unit. JAMA 2004;291: 1753–62.
23. Lin SM, Liu CY, Wang CH, et al. The impact of delirium on the survival of mechanically ventilated patients. Crit Care Med 2004;32:2254–9.
24. Buurman BM, Hoogerduijn JG, de Haan RJ, et al. Geriatric conditions in acutely hospitalized older patients: prevalence and one-year survival and functional decline. PLoS One 2011;6:e26951.
25. Pitkala KH, Laurila JV, Strandberg TE, et al. Prognostic significance of delirium in frail older people. Dement Geriatr Cogn Disord 2005;19:158–63.
26. Leslie DL, Zhang Y, Holford TR, et al. Premature death associated with delirium at 1-year follow-up. Arch Intern Med 2005;165:1657–62.
27. Han JH, Shintani A, Eden S, et al. Delirium in the emergency department: an independent predictor of death within 6 months. Ann Emerg Med 2010;56: 244–52.

28. Hatherill S, Flisher AJ. Delirium in children and adolescents: a systematic review of the literature. J Psychosom Res 2010;68(4):337–44. Available at: http://documentslide. com/documents/delirium-in-children-and-adolescents-a-systematic-review-of-the-literature.html.

29. SantaCruz KS, Sonnen JA, Pezhouh MK, et al. Alzheimer's disease pathology in subjects without dementia in 2 studies of aging: the Nun study and the Adult Changes in Thought Study. J Neuropathol Exp Neurol 2011;70(10): 832–40.

30. Iacono D, Markesbery WR, Gross M, et al. The Nun study: clinically silent AD, neuronal hypertrophy, and linguistic skills in early life. Neurology 2009;73(9): 665–73.

31. Jones RN, Fong TG, Metzger E, et al. Aging, brain disease, and reserve: implications for delirium. Am J Geriatr Psychiatry 2010;18:117–27.

32. Izaks GI, Westendorp RG. Ill or just old? Towards a conceptual framework of the relation between ageing and disease. BMC Geriatr 2003;3:7.

33. Davis DHJ, Muniz-Terrera G, Keage AD, et al. Association of delirium with cognitive decline in late life: a neuropathological study of 3 population-based cohort studies. JAMA Psychiatry 2017. http://dx.doi.org/10.1001/jamapsychiatry.2016. 3423.

34. Wilson RS, Hebert LE, Scherr PA, et al. Cognitive decline after hospitalization in a community population of older persons. Neurology 2012;78:950–6.

35. Solberg LM, Plummer CE, May KN, et al. 'A quality improvement program to increase nurses' detection of delirium on an acute medical unit. Geriatr Nurs 2013;34(1):75.

36. Saczynski JS, Marcantonio ER, Quach L, et al. Cognitive trajectories after postoperative delirium. N Engl J Med 2012;367:30–9.

37. Davis DH, Muniz Terrera G, Keage H, et al. Delirium is a strong risk factor for dementia in the oldest-old: a population-based cohort study. Brain 2012;135: 2809–16.

38. Pandharipande PP, Girard TD, Jackson JC, et al. Long-term cognitive impairment after critical illness. N Engl J Med 2013;369(14):1306–16.

39. Wong CL, Holroyd-Leduc J, Simel JD, et al. Does this patient have delirium?: value of bedside instruments. JAMA 2010;304:779–86.

40. Gaudreau JD, Gagnon P, Harel F, et al. Fast, systematic, and continuous delirium assessment in hospitalized patients: the nursing delirium screening scale. J Pain Symptom Manage 2005;29:368–75.

41. Schuurmans MJ, Shortridge-Baggett LM, Duursma SA. The delirium observation screening scale: a screening instrument for delirium. Res Theory Nurs Pract 2003;17:31–50.

42. Neelon VJ, Champagne MT, Carlson JR, et al. The NEECHAM confusion scale: construction, validation, and clinical testing. Nurs Res 1996;45:324–30.

43. Inouye SK, van Dyck CH, Alessi CA, et al. Clarifying confusion: the confusion assessment method. A new method for detection of delirium. Ann Intern Med 1990;113:941–8.

44. De J, Wand AP, Smerdely PI, et al. Validating the 4A's test in screening for delirium in a culturally diverse geriatric inpatient population. Int J Geriatr Psychiatry 2016. [Epub ahead of print].

45. Wei LA, Fearing MA, Sternberg EJ, et al. The confusion assessment method: a systematic review of current usage. J Am Geriatr Soc 2008;56:823–30.

46. Inouye SK. The short confusion assessment method (Short CAM): training manual and coding guide. Boston: Hospital Elder life Program; 2014.

47. Ely EW, Margolin R, Francis J, et al. Evaluation of delirium in critically ill patients: validation of the confusion assessment method for the intensive care unit (CAM-ICU). Crit Care Med 2011;29:1370–9.

48. Han JH, Wilson A, Graves AJ, et al. Validation of the confusion assessment method for the intensive care unit in older emergency department patients. Acad Emerg Med 2014;21(2):180–7.

49. Ely EW, Stephens RK, Jackson JC, et al. Current opinions regarding the importance, diagnosis, and management of delirium in the intensive care unit: a survey of 912 healthcare professionals. Crit Care Med 2004;32(1):106–12.

50. Han JH, Zimmerman EE, Cutler N. Delirium in older emergency department patients: recognition, risk factors, and psychomotor subtypes. Acad Emerg Med 2009;16(3):193–200.

51. Collins N, Blanchard MR, Tookman A, et al. Detection of delirium in the acute hospital. Age Ageing 2010;39(1):131–5.

52. Marcantonio ED. In the clinic. Delirium. Ann Intern Med 2011;154:ITC6-1-15.

53. Mrak RE, Griffin WST. Dementia with Lewy bodies: definition, diagnosis, and pathological relationship to Alzheimer's disease. Neuropsychiatr Dis Treat 2007; 3(5):619–25.

54. Hughes CG, Patel MB, Pandharipande PP. Pathophysiology of acute brain dysfunction: what's the cause of all this confusion? Curr Opin Crit Care 2012; 18(5):518–26.

55. Choi SH, Lee H, Chung TS, et al. Neural network functional connectivity during and after an episode of delirium. Am J Psychiatry 2012;169:498–507.

56. Lauretani F, Ceda GP, Maggio M, et al. Capturing side-effect of medication to identify persons at risk of delirium. Aging Clin Exp Res 2010;22:456–8.

57. Hshieh TT, Fong TG, Marcantonio ER, et al. Cholinergic deficiency hypothesis in delirium: a synthesis of current evidence. J Gerontol A Biol Sci Med Sci 2008;63: 764–72.

58. Risacher SL, McDonald BC, Tallman EF, et al, Alzheimer's Disease Neuroimaging Initiative. Association between anticholinergic medication use and cognition, brain metabolism, and brain atrophy in cognitively normal older adults. JAMA Neurol 2016;73(6):721–32.

59. Gaudreau JD, Gagnon P. Psychotogenic drugs and delirium pathogenesis: the central role of the thalamus. Med Hypotheses 2005;64:471–5.

60. Young BK, Camicioli R, Ganzini L. Neuropsychiatric adverse effects of antiparkinsonian drugs. Characteristics, evaluation and treatment. Drugs Aging 1997;10: 367–83.

61. Alagiakrishnan K, Wiens CA. An approach to drug induced delirium in the elderly. Postgrad Med J 2004;80:388–93.

62. Maclullich AM, Ferguson KJ, Miller T, et al. Unravelling the pathophysiology of delirium: a focus on the role of aberrant stress responses. J Psychosom Res 2008;65:229–38.

63. Schoen J, Meyerrose J, Paarmann H, et al. Preoperative regional cerebral oxygen saturation is a predictor of postoperative delirium in on-pump cardiac surgery patients: a prospective observational trial. Crit Care 2011; 15:R218.

64. Joels M. Impact of glucocorticoids on brain function: relevance for mood disorders. Psychoneuroendocrinology 2011;36:406–14.

65. Marcantonio ER, Rudolph JL, Culley D, et al. Serum biomarkers for delirium. J Gerontol A Biol Sci Med Sci 2006;61:1281–6.

66. Dantzer R, O'Connor JC, Freund GG, et al. From inflammation to sickness and depression: when the immune system subjugates the brain. Nat Rev Neurosci 2008;9:46–56.

67. Stagno D Jr, Gibson C Jr, Breitbart W Jr. The delirium subtypes: a review of prevalence, phenomenology, pathophysiology, and treatment response. Palliat Support Care 2004;2(2):171.

68. Cunningham C, Campion S, Lunnon K, et al. Systemic inflammation induces acute behavioral and cognitive changes and accelerates neurodegenerative disease. Biol Psychiatry 2009;65:304–12.

69. Cunningham C. Systemic inflammation and delirium: important co-factors in the progression of dementia. Biochem Soc Trans 2011;39:945–53.

70. van Gool WA, van de Beek D, Eikelenboom P. Systemic infection and delirium: when cytokines and acetylcholine collide. Lancet 2010;375:773–5.

71. Zampieri FG, Park M, Machado FS, et al. Sepsis-associated encephalopathy: not just delirium. Clinics (Sao Paulo) 2011;66:1825–31.

72. Flaherty JH, Gonzales JP, Dong B. Antipsychotics in the treatment of delirium in older hospitalized adults: a systemic review. J Am Geriatr Soc 2011;59(Suppl 2): S269–76.

73. Page VJ, Ely EW, Gates S, et al. Effect of intravenous haloperidol on the duration of delirium and coma in critically ill patients (Hope-ICU): a randomized, double-blind, placebo-controlled trail. Lancet Respir Med 2013;1(7).515–23.

74. Morandi A, Davis D, Taylor JK, et al. Consensus and variations in opinions on delirium care: a survey of European delirium specialists. Int Psychogeriatr 2013;25(12):2067–75.

75. Barr J, Fraser GL, Puntillo K, et al. Clinical practice guidelines for the management of pain, agitation and delirium in adult patients in the intensive care unit. Crit Care Med 2013;4(1):278–80.

76. Barr J, Pandharipande PP. The pain, agitation, and delirium care bundle: synergistic benefits of implementing the 2013 pain, agitation, and delirium guidelines in an integrated and interdisciplinary fashion. Crit Care Med 2013;41(9):S99–115.

77. Martin S, Fernandees L. Delirium in elderly people: a review. Front Neurol 2012;3:101.

78. Tabet N, Hudson S, Sweeney V, et al. An educational intervention can prevent delirium on acute medical wards. Age Ageing 2005;34(2):152–6.

79. Maldonado JR. Pathoetiological model of delirium: a comprehensive understanding of the neurobiology of delirium and an evidence-based approach to prevention and treatment. Crit Care Clin 2008;24:789–856.

80. American Geriatrics Society 2015 Beers Criteria Update Expert Panel. American Geriatrics Society 2015 updated Beers criteria for potentially inappropriate medication use in older adults. J Am Geriatr Soc 2015;63:2227–46.

81. Boustani MA, Campbell NL, Munger S, et al. Impact of anticholinergics on the aging brain: a review and practical application. Aging Health 2008;4(3):311–20.

82. Schaller SJ, Anstey M, Blobner M, et al. Early, goal-directed mobilisation in the surgical intensive care unit: a randomised controlled trial. Lancet 2016; 388(10052):1377–88.

83. Campbell N, Boustani M, Limbil T, et al. The cognitive impact of anticholinergics: a clinical review. Clin Interv Aging 2009;4(1):225–33.

84. Clegg A, Young J, Illiffe S, et al. Frailty in elderly people. Lancet 2013;381(9868): 752–62.

85. Vasilevskis EE, Ely EW. 2013: updates in delirium. Neurohospitalist 2014;4(2): 58–60.

86. National Institute for Health and Clinical Excellence. 2010. Available at: www.nice. org.uk/cg103. Accessed February 10, 2017.

87. Aquirre E. Delirium and hospitalized older adults: a review of non-pharmacological treatment. J Contin Educ Nurs 2010;41(4):151–2.

88. Brown TM, Boyle MF. Delirium. BMJ 2002;325(7365):644.

APPENDIX 1: 4-AT DELIRIUM ASSESSMENT

(label)

4AT

**Assessment test
for delirium &
cognitive impairment**

Patient name:

Date of birth:

Patient number:

Date: Time:

Tester:

	CIRCLE

[1] ALERTNESS
This includes patients who may be markedly drowsy (eg, difficult to rouse and/or obviously sleepy during assessment) or agitated/hyperactive. Observe the patient. If asleep, attempt to wake with speech or gentle touch on shoulder. Ask the patient to state their name and address to assist rating.

Normal (fully alert, but not agitated, throughout assessment)	0
Mild sleepiness for <10 s after waking, then normal	0
Clearly abnormal	4

[2] AMT4
Age, date of birth, place (name of the hospital or building), current year.

No mistakes	0
1 mistake	1
2 or more mistakes/untestable	2

[3] ATTENTION
*Ask the patient: "Please tell me the months of the year in backwards order, starting at December."
To assist initial understanding one prompt of "what is the month before December?" is permitted.*

Months of the year backwards		
	Achieves 7 mo or more correctly	0
	Starts but scores <7 mo / refuses to start	1
	Untestable (cannot start because unwell, drowsy, inattentive)	2

[4] ACUTE CHANGE OR FLUCTUATING COURSE
Evidence of significant change or fluctuation in: alertness, cognition, other mental function (eg, paranoia, hallucinations) arising over the last 2 wk and still evident in last 24 h

No	0
Yes	4

4 or above: possible delirium +/- cognitive impairment
1–3: possible cognitive impairment
0: delirium or severe cognitive impairment unlikely (but delirium still possible if [4] information incomplete)

4AT SCORE [   ]

GUIDANCE NOTES   Version 1.2. Information and download: www.the4AT.com
The 4AT is a screening instrument designed for rapid initial assessment of delirium and cognitive impairment. A score of 4 or more *suggests* delirium but is not diagnostic: more detailed assessment of mental status may be required to reach a diagnosis. A score of 1-3 suggests cognitive impairment and more detailed cognitive testing and informant history-taking are required. A score of 0 does not definitively exclude delirium or cognitive impairment: more detailed testing may be required depending on the clinical context. Items 1-3 are rated *solely on observation of the patient at the time of assessment.* Item 4 requires information from one or more source(s), eg, your own knowledge of the patient, other staff who know the patient (eg, ward nurses), GP letter, case notes, carers. The tester should take account of communication difficulties (hearing impairment, dysphasia, lack of common language) when carrying out the test and interpreting the score.
Alertness: Altered level of alertness is very likely to be delirium in general hospital settings. If the patient shows significant altered alertness during the bedside assessment, score 4 for this item. **AMT4 (Abbreviated Mental Test - 4):** This score can be extracted from items in the AMT10 if the latter is done immediately before. **Acute Change or Fluctuating Course:** Fluctuation can occur without delirium in some cases of dementia, but marked fluctuation usually indicates delirium. To help elicit any hallucinations and/or paranoid thoughts ask the patient questions such as, "Are you concerned about anything going on here?"; "Do you feel frightened by anything or anyone?"; "Have you been seeing or hearing anything unusual?"

APPENDIX 2: SCOTTISH DELIRIUM ASSOCIATION DELIRIUM MANAGEMENT PATHWAY FOR CARE HOMES

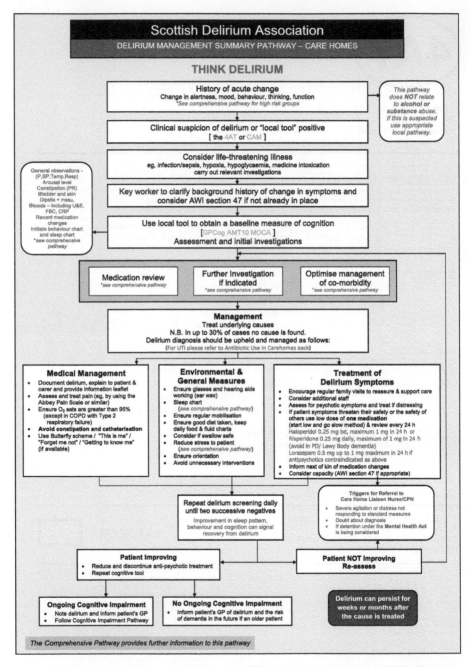

From Scottish Delirium Association. Available at: http://www.scottishdelirium association.com/. Accessed February 10, 2017; with permission.

APPENDIX 3: SCOTTISH DELIRIUM ASSOCIATION COMPREHENSIVE DELIRIUM PATHWAY

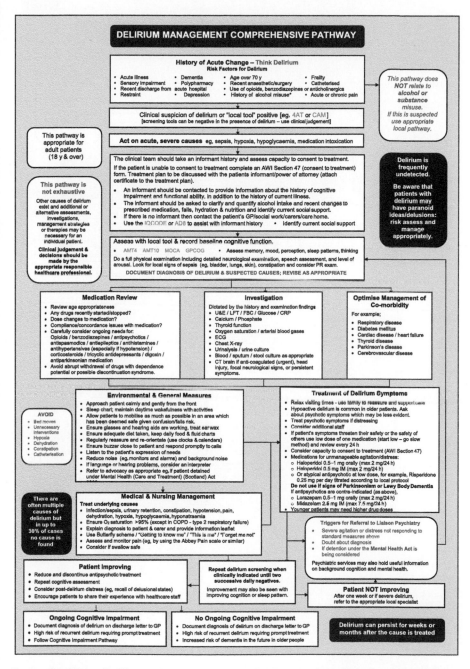

From Scottish Delirium Association. Available at: http://www.scottishdelirium association.com/. Accessed February 10, 2017; with permission.

Moving?

Make sure your subscription moves with you!

To notify us of your new address, find your **Clinics Account Number** (located on your mailing label above your name), and contact customer service at:

Email: journalscustomerservice-usa@elsevier.com

800-654-2452 (subscribers in the U.S. & Canada)
314-447-8871 (subscribers outside of the U.S. & Canada)

Fax number: 314-447-8029

Elsevier Health Sciences Division
Subscription Customer Service
3251 Riverport Lane
Maryland Heights, MO 63043

*To ensure uninterrupted delivery of your subscription, please notify us at least 4 weeks in advance of move.

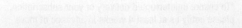